Understand your diabetes...

AND LIVE A HEALTHY LIFE

Understand your diabetes...

AND LIVE A HEALTHY LIFE

Diabetes Day Care Unit, Hôtel-Dieu of the Health Center
of the University of Montreal

GLOBALMEDIC

Rogers Media

Canadian Cataloguing in Publication Data

Main entry under title:

Understand your diabetes... and live a healthy life

Translation of the 3rd ed. of: Connaître son diabète... pour mieux vivre!
"GlobalMedic"

ISBN 2-922260-08-9

1.Diabetes – Popular works. 2. Diabetics – Health and hygiene. 3. Diabetes – Diet therapy.
I. Université de Montréal. Centre hospitalier universitaire. Pavillon Hôtel-Dieu. Unité de jour de diabète.

RC660.4.C6613 2001   616.4'62   C2001-941514-1

Legal deposit: 4th quarter 2001
Bibliothèque nationale du Québec
National Library of Canada

◆ ROGERS

www.lactualite.com/livres

The publication of this work was made possible thanks to unrestricted grants
from Pfizer Canada Inc. and Aventis Pharma.

 Aventis Pharma

Life is our life's work

Translation: Ovid Da Silva
Graphics conception and cover design: Pascal Gornick

Printed in Canada

Preface

For those of you new to the diagnosis of diabetes and to those of you who are taking the steps required to ensure an active and productive life as a person with diabetes, this publication is an effort to support you. There has never been a more challenging time in diabetes as new medications, new technologies and new information transform our understanding of how to better care, manage and treat diabetes in Canada.

Diabetes care hinges on the daily commitment of the person with diabetes to make healthy choices. The information contained within this book is an excellent resource aimed at assisting the person with diabetes to live a healthy lifestyle and strive for glucose levels that will assist in the delay and/or prevention of both long and short-term complications of diabetes. The Canadian Diabetes Association's mission to promote the health of Canadians through diabetes research, education, service and advocacy recognizes the importance of resources such as this publication to assist the person with diabetes. On behalf of the Association, I applaud the authors' edition of *Understand Your Diabetes… And Live a Healthy Life*.

Jim O'Brien, Chief Executive Officer,
Canadian Diabetes Association

Foreword

Our understanding of diabetes, the diagnosis of the disease, its causes, its complications, and, above all, its treatment are constantly evolving. It is, therefore, important for people with diabetes to be better informed. This will allow them to take charge of their diabetes and increase their chances of gaining optimal control of the disease – and, thus, avoid short- and long-term complications.

This edition features a great deal of new and practical information that will help the general population and, especially, people with diabetes. We have, for example, presented some statistics on the growing problem of diabetes in the world, and we have included new criteria for the diagnosis of the disease. We have updated the list of devices for measuring capillary blood glucose (blood sugar) that are increasingly easy to use and thus carry less risk of errors. Two new antidiabetic medications have been added to the list: Avandia® and Actos®, which are members of a new family of medications, the thiazolidinediones, that increase the action of insulin. We have similarly included a new insulin that has just arrived on the market: Humalog® Mix 25, a premixed insulin. At the nutritional level, we thought it would be appropriate to explain the different modes of expression of carbohydrates (sugars) in food. We have likewise included a table illustrating the main effects of fats and other factors on blood lipids. Finally, we have insisted on the psychological aspect to better define the relationship between depression, anxiety and diabetes.

We hope that this book will help people with diabetes to better understand their disease and provide a tool to improve their condition and maintain a better quality of life.

The Team of the Diabetes Day Care Unit,
Hôtel-Dieu of the Health Center of the University of Montreal

Authors

This work was achieved by the members of the Multidisciplinary Team of the Diabetes Day Care Unit, Hôtel-Dieu of the Health Center of the University of Montreal:

- Dr. Jean-Louis Chiasson, Endocrinologist

- Nathalie Beaulieu, Dietitian

- Françoise Desrochers, Registered Nurse, B.Sc.

- Sylvie Fournier, Pharmacist

- Lyne Gauthier, Pharmacist

- Christiane Gobeil, Dietitian

- Michelle Messier, Dietitian

- Nicole Hamel, Pharmacist

- Charles Tourigny, Psychologist

Acknowledgements

We thank the members of the Endocrinology, Metabolism and Nutrition Division, Hôtel-Dieu of the Health Center of the University of Montreal, for their contribution. We also thank Susanne Bordeleau-Chénier for her invaluable secretarial work.

Objectives of this book

General objective

To help people with diabetes optimally improve their health status and reduce the number of hospitalizations as well as the short- and long-term complications associated with diabetes.

Specific objectives

To help people with diabetes adopt lifestyle habits that are conducive to the maintenance of normal blood glucose levels and to make them capable of:

1) acquiring general knowledge on diabetes;

2) adapting their diet according to their diabetes and their different activities;

3) taking into account the influence of stress and physical exercise on the control of their disease;

4) knowing the complications caused by variations in blood glucose levels;

5) effectively intervening during the manifestations of complications;

6) administering medications adequately;

7) understanding the importance of caring for their feet;

8) adequately manipulating devices that measure capillary blood glucose;

9) using community resources according to their needs.

Table of contents

Chapter 1
General information on diabetes

1. What is diabetes?

Diabetes is a disease characterized by an **elevation of the blood glucose or blood sugar level** that is above normal.

2. How many Canadians are affected by diabetes?

Diabetes affects about **two million Canadians** (7% of the population), but nearly half of them have not yet been diagnosed and are not aware of their condition. It is anticipated that the number of diagnosed cases will double by the year 2010, making diabetes the **disease of the 21st century**.

Constituting an increasingly heavy economic burden to Canada, presently estimated to be nearly **10 billion dollars** per year in direct and indirect costs, diabetes is a growing societal problem that must be combatted on all fronts.

3. What are the criteria for diagnosing diabetes?

The diagnosis of diabetes is based on the results of tests done on venous blood and include:

1) **a fasting blood glucose level** higher than or equal to 7.0 mmol/L; or,

2) **a random blood glucose level** higher than or equal to 11.1 mmol/L; or,

3) **a glucose tolerance test with a blood glucose level:** Higher than or equal to 11.1 mmol/L two hours after the consumption of 75 g of glucose.

However, to establish the diagnosis of diabetes, an abnormal value of any one of these tests must be confirmed a second time, on another day, by repeating anyone of these tests.

4. What is a normal or optimal blood glucose level?

In people with diabetes, the blood glucose level is considered "normal" as long as it stays between **4 and 7 mmol/L before meals, and between 5 and 11 mmol/L one to two hours after meals**.

5. What is the cause of diabetes?

Diabetes is caused by a **lack of insulin**.

6. Where does insulin come from?

Insulin is produced by the **pancreas**, an organ located in the abdomen, behind the stomach.

7. What is glucose used for in the body?

Glucose is an important **source of energy** for cells of the body, in the same way as gas is the source of energy for a car.

8. What is insulin used for in the body?

We could say that insulin is the **key that allows glucose to enter the cells**, just like an ignition key is used to start a car. By letting glucose enter the cells, insulin lowers the blood glucose level.

9. Why does the blood glucose level rise in a diabetic person?

In people with diabetes, the **pancreas does not produce enough insulin** to allow glucose to enter the cells. As a result, the blood glucose level rises. This is called hyperglycemia.

10. Where does the excess glucose found in the blood of diabetic persons come from?

Blood glucose comes from two sources:

1) **foods containing carbohydrates (sugars)** consumed at meal time and by snacking;

2) the **liver**, which stores the glucose at meal time and releases it subsequently into the blood between meals.

11. What are the characteristics of type 1 diabetes?

Type 1 diabetes is generally characterized by the following factors:

1) the **total absence of insulin**;

2) its appearance towards **puberty** and **before the age of 40 years**;

3) **weight loss**;

4) the need for treatment with **insulin injections**.

12. What are the characteristics of type 2 diabetes?

Type 2 diabetes is generally characterized by the following factors:

1) the pancreas produces insulin but in **insufficient quantity** and the insulin produced is less effective – this is called **insulin resistance**;

2) it generally appears **after the age of 40 years**;

3) **excess weight**;

4) the need for treatment with a **dietary program** alone or with **oral antidiabetic medications**, and sometimes with **insulin injections**.

13. What is the goal of diabetes treatment?

The goal of diabetes treatment is to lower and **maintain the blood glucose level as close to normal as possible**.

14. Why is it so important to have a normal blood glucose level?

A normal blood glucose level allows a diabetic person:

1) to feel in **better shape**;

2) to avoid the long-term **complications** related to diabetes.

15. How can a diabetic person reach and maintain a normal blood glucose level?

To control your diabetes, it is important to **take charge** of your disease and follow these guidelines:

1) respect the **prescribed dietary plan** and aim for a normal weight;

2) **exercise** regularly;

3) measure your **capillary blood glucose level** regularly;

4) take your antidiabetic **medications as** prescribed;

5) **adapt** to the disease and learn to **manage** stress;

6) be well **informed** about diabetes.

- **You are the person who is best placed, in collaboration with the team of professionals, to control your diabetes.**

- **Diabetes is a chronic disease which cannot be cured, but can be controlled.**

- **You have done nothing to have diabetes.**

- **The more you are capable of keeping your blood glucose level as close to normal as possible, the better you will feel.**

- **Keeping yourself informed about diabetes will give you a better chance to control it.**

Notes

Chapter 2
Hyperglycemia

1. What is hyperglycemia?

Hyperglycemia is an increase in **the blood glucose level above normal**, that is, above 7 mmol/L before meals and above 11 mmol/L one or two hours after meals.

2. Why do people with diabetes develop hyperglycemia?

People with diabetes develop hyperglycemia when **the amount of insulin in the blood is insufficient compared to the amount of glucose being released in the blood**.

3. What are the symptoms of hyperglycemia?

When blood glucose rises above a certain level, the following symptoms may appear:

1) **increase in the volume and frequency of urine**;

2) intense **thirst**;

3) exaggerated **hunger**;

4) **weight loss**.

Hyperglycemia can also be associated with:

5) **blurred vision**;

6) **infections**, especially of the genital organs and bladder;

7) **wounds** that heal poorly;

8) **fatigue**;

9) **sleepiness**;

10) **irritability**.

4. What are the main causes of hyperglycemia?

The principal causes of hyperglycemia are:

1) an increase in food intake **containing carbohydrates (sugars)**;

2) **decreased physical activity**;

3) **incorrect dosage** of antidiabetic medications (insulin or pills);

4) an **infection**;

5) too much **stress**;

6) taking certain **medications** such as glucocorticoids (e.g. cortisone);

7) **nocturnal hypoglycemia** followed by a **hyperglycemic rebound in the morning**.

5. What must a diabetic do when hyperglycemia is suspected?

When someone suspects he/she has hyperglycemia, it is important to do the following:

1) **measure his/her capillary blood glucose**;

2) if the blood glucose is higher than 15 mmol/L, people with type 1 diabetes must **verify the presence of ketone bodies** in urine;

3) **drink a lot of water** to avoid dehydration;

4) identify the cause of hyperglycemia;

5) correct the cause if possible;

6) call the doctor or go to emergency:

   ■ if blood glucose is above 20 mmol/L;

   ■ if the presence of ketone bodies in urine is from average to high;

   ■ if it is impossible to retain liquids taken orally.

6. What are the long-term complications of hyperglycemia?

In the long-term, hyperglycemia can lead to complications of the eyes, kidneys, nerves, heart and blood vessels.

Notes

Chapter 3
Hypoglycemia and glucagon

1. What is hypoglycemia?

Hypoglycemia is a fall in the blood glucose level **below normal**, that is, below 4 mmol/L.

2. Why does hypoglycemia occur?

Hypoglycemia occurs when there is **too much insulin** in the blood for the amount of glucose present.

3. Who is susceptible to hypoglycemia?

People **injecting themselves with insulin** or **taking medications which stimulate the pancreas to produce more insulin**, such as chlorpropamide (Diabinese®), tolbutamide (Mobenol®, Orinase®), glyburide (Diaßeta®, Euglucon®), gliclazide (Diamicron®) and repaglinide (GlucoNorm®), are susceptible to experience hypoglycemia.

4. What are the signs of hypoglycemia?

If hypoglycemia appears **rapidly**, it can produce the following symptoms:

1) **tremor**;

2) **palpitations**;

3) **sweating or perspiration**;

4) **blurred vision**;

5) **dizziness**;

6) **paleness**;

7) **acute hunger**;

8) **weakness**;

9) **nightmares and agitated sleep if hypoglycemia occurs during sleep**;

10) **morning hyperglycemia** following nocturnal hypoglycemia: awakening in a sweat and with a headache.

If hypoglycemia appears **slowly**, the signs are more discreet:

1) **numbness around the mouth**;

2) **yawning**;

3) **fatigue**;

4) **urge to sleep**;

5) **mood change**;

6) **aggressiveness**;

7) **confusion**.

If the hypoglycemia is not reversed, it can cause **loss of consciousness**.

5. What causes hypoglycemia?

The most frequent causes of hypoglycemia are:

1) **incorrect dosage** of antidiabetic medications (insulin or pills);

2) **a skipped snack or meal**;

3) **a delayed meal**;

4) eating a **smaller than necessary quantity of food containing carbohydrates (sugars)**;

5) **an error** in evaluating the level of carbohydrates in food;

6) **increased physical activity**;

7) **alcohol consumption**;

8) an overtreatment of high blood glucose with rapid or short acting insulin.

6. What should people with diabetes do when hypoglycemia is suspected?

When a diabetic suspects hypoglycemia, he/she should not go to bed without treating the hypoglycemia, thinking that the blood glucose level will correct itself. He/she must immediately:

1) **measure his/her capillary blood glucose level**;

2) **eat food that supplies** about 15 g of carbohydrates, preferably food that is quickly absorbed such as:

   ■ 3 tablets of Glucose BD® (1 tablet = 5 g of carbohydrates)

- 5 tablets of Dextrosol® (1 tablet = 3 g of carbohydrates)

- 125 mL (4 ounces) of fruit juice

- 125 mL (4 ounces) of a regular soft drink

- 15 mL (3 teaspoons) of sugar dissolved in water

- 15 mL (3 teaspoons) of honey, jam, syrup

- 6 Life Saver® candies

- 250 mL (1 cup) of milk

- 200 mL (1 carton) of milk, plus 2 dry "Social Tea" biscuits

- 4 dry "Social Tea" biscuits

> **In people with diabetes who take Acarbose (Prandase®), hypoglycemia must be corrected, preferably with three tablets of Glucose BD® or with milk (250 mL).**

3) **avoid overtreatment:**

- **wait 20 minutes, measure the blood glucose level again**;

- take an additional 15 g of carbohydrates if the hypoglycemia persists.

After correcting the hypoglycemia, if you have to wait more than two hours for the next meal, it is often recommended to add a snack containing 15 g of carbohydrates (e.g. 250 mL of milk, or 6 to 8 crackers + cheese, or fruit + cheese).

4) **try to identify the cause**.

7. Why is it important to treat hypoglycemia immediately?

It is important to treat hypoglycemia **immediately** because of the risk of **coma** which could follow.

8. How can hypoglycemia be avoided?

Hypoglycemia can generally be avoided if the following precautions are taken:

1) measure **your capillary blood glucose** regularly;

2) **carefully follow the dietary program** prescription, including meal distribution, snacks and their carbohydrate content;

3) have a **bedtime snack** if it is part of your dietary prescription;

4) carefully follow the **advice of your doctor and the dietitian** before beginning exercise or physical activity;

5) avoid consuming **alcohol on an empty stomach**;

6) if needed, check your blood glucose level around **2 a.m.**

9. What precautions should be taken to avoid potential accidents due to hypoglycemia?

1) **always have a food that contains glucose with you**;

2) wear **a bracelet or a pendant** which identifies you as a diabetic;

3) **warn** your family, friends and colleagues at work that you are diabetic. Describe to them the signs of hypoglycemia and how they can help you to correct it;

4) if you are on insulin, always have **glucagon** within reach at home, at work or when travelling. A close relative or someone you know well must learn how to inject it in case you develop severe hypoglycemia.

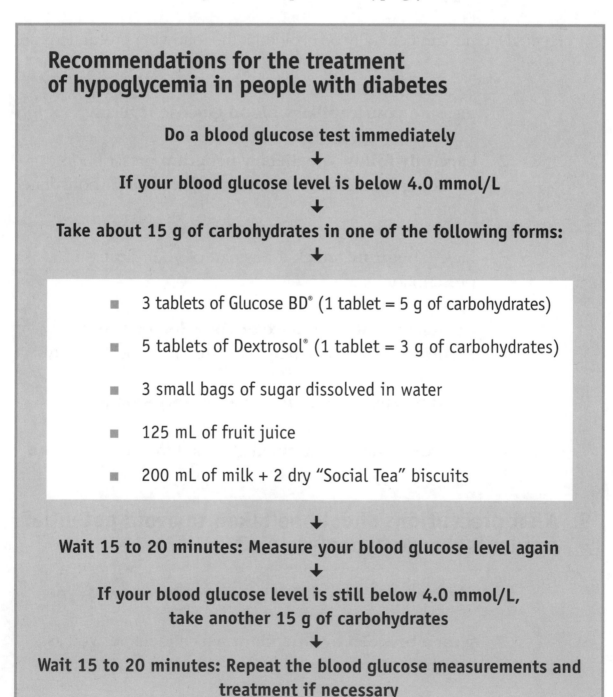

Recommendations for the treatment of hypoglycemia in people with diabetes

Do a blood glucose test immediately

↓

If your blood glucose level is below 4.0 mmol/L

↓

Take about 15 g of carbohydrates in one of the following forms:

↓

- 3 tablets of Glucose BD® (1 tablet = 5 g of carbohydrates)

- 5 tablets of Dextrosol® (1 tablet = 3 g of carbohydrates)

- 3 small bags of sugar dissolved in water

- 125 mL of fruit juice

- 200 mL of milk + 2 dry "Social Tea" biscuits

↓

Wait 15 to 20 minutes: Measure your blood glucose level again

↓

If your blood glucose level is still below 4.0 mmol/L, take another 15 g of carbohydrates

↓

Wait 15 to 20 minutes: Repeat the blood glucose measurements and treatment if necessary

When the blood glucose level is higher than or equal to 4.0 mmol/L
↓

Meal (or snack) expected within the next two hours?

↓ | ↓
Yes | **No**
Take it as usual | Add a snack containing 15 g
 | of carbohydrates
 | Example: Milk (200 mL) +
 | 2 dry "Social Tea" biscuits

Warning

1. In people with diabetes who take **Acarbose** (Prandase®), hypoglycemia must be corrected preferably with 15 g of glucose:

   ■ 3 tablets of Glucose BD®

   ■ 250 mL of milk

2. In people with diabetes suffering from **kidney problems**, it is advisable to correct hypoglycemia in one of the following ways:

   ■ 3 tablets of Glucose BD® (1 tablet = 5 g of carbohydrates)

   ■ 5 tablets of Dextrosol® (1 tablet = 3 g of carbohydrates)

   ■ 3 small bags of sugar dissolved in water

3. After a **severe hypoglycemic episode** (requiring the help of another person), if the diabetic was given a glucagon injection, a substantial snack containing 45 g of carbohydrates — sandwich + milk (200 mL) — should be provided as soon as he/she recovers consciousness.

Notes

Chapter 4
Self-monitoring: Capillary blood glucose and glycosylated hemoglobin

1. What is self-monitoring of blood glucose?

Self-monitoring of blood glucose is a technique used by the diabetic person to **measure his/her own blood glucose level**. In a broader sense, this approach generally includes the **adjustment** of treatment according to the results in order to bring and maintain the blood glucose level as close to normal as possible.

2. Why should people with diabetes practise self-monitoring of blood glucose?

Self-monitoring of blood glucose is meant to:

1) check the impact of **nutrition**, **physical exercise**, antidiabetic medication and stress on blood glucose;

2) identify any **hypoglycemia and hyperglycemia** in order to take rapid action;

3) **change behavior** concerning nutrition, physical exercise, antidiabetic medication and stress;

4) check the impact of these **adjustments** on blood glucose;

5) develop a feeling of confidence and security as well as the capacity to control your own diabetes; and, especially,

6) **bring and maintain the blood glucose level as close to normal as possible**.

3. Why should people with diabetes try to maintain normal blood glucose values?

If possible, people with diabetes should always try to maintain a "normal" blood glucose level, that is, **between 4 and 7 mmol/L before meals** and **between 5 and 11 mmol/L one to two hours after meals**, to prevent complications associated with diabetes.

Two major studies, one American in type 1 diabetes, and the other British in type 2 diabetes, showed that keeping blood glucose close to normal **significantly reduced the appearance and progression of diabetic complications**:

- **Retinopathy**: ↓ 27 to 76%

- **Nephropathy**: ↓ 34 to 57%

- **Neuropathy**: ↓ 60%

4. How is the blood glucose level measured?

Capillary blood glucose is measured in two steps:

Preparing the material and checking the test strips

1) **Wash your hands** with soapy water and dry them thoroughly.

2) Prepare **the material**: reader, test strip, holder, lancet, paper tissue.

3) Insert the lancet into the **holder** and set it.

4) Check the **expiry dates** on the packaging of the test strip (the expiry date assigned by the manufacturer and the expiry date recorded by you on opening the container).

5) Take out a **test strip**. If the strip comes from a bottle, close it immediately.

Blood analysis and data recording

1) Press on the switch of the monitoring device to start it.

2) Insert the test strip in the strip support of the device.

3) Prick the **lateral extremity** of a finger (change fingers each time).

4) Make a **large drop of blood** come out of the finger by putting pressure on it and holding it downwards.

5) Depending on the device used, lay the drop of blood on the reactive part of the strip or bring the reactive part of the strip into contact with the blood.

6) Wait for the reading to be displayed.

7) **Write the result** in the appropriate column of your logbook.

5. What capillary glucose meters are available and what are their features?

Here is a list of capillary glucose meters found on the market, with some of their features (list revised as of February 1, 2001):

Capillary glucose meters cost between $0 and $100, depending on the model. Often, there are promotions, and some devices are free if exchanged for a used one.

The strips cost between $0.90 and $1.00. There are never any promotions for the strips.

Name	Glucometer® Elite®	Glucometer® Elite® XL	Glucometer® Dex®	One Touch® Profile®	Sure Step®
Manufacturer	**Bayer**	**Bayer**	**Bayer**	**LifeScan**	**LifeScan**
1. Measuring range (mmol/L)	1.1 to 33.3	1.1 to 33.3	0.6 to 33.3	0 to 33.3	0 to 27.8
2. Duration of analysis (seconds)	30	30	30	45	30
3. Memory	20	120	100	250	10
4. Connection to a PC	No	Yes (memory: 120)	Yes (memory: 100)	Yes (memory: 250)	Yes (memory: 150)
5. Cleaning required	No	No	No	Yes	Yes
6. Quality control of meters	CHECK calibration strip	CHECK calibration strip	Automatic calibration	Purple calibration strip	Automatic calibration
7. Calibration of test strips	Calibration strip in each box	Calibration strip in each box	Automatic calibration	Calibration code on each bottle	Calibration code on each bottle
8. Quantity of blood required	2 µL	2 µL	3 µL	10 µL	10 µL
9. Possibility of adding a 2nd drop of blood	No	No	No	No	Yes (confirmation point)
10. Test strips	Packed separately	Packed separately	Disk of 10 strips	In a bottle (sensitive to humidity)	In a bottle (sensitive to humidity)
11. Can the test strip be touched?	Yes	Yes	Yes	No	Yes
12. Lifespan of the test strips	1 year (date printed on packet)	1 year (date printed on packet)	2 years (date printed on disk)	4 months	4 months
13. Control solution, conservation time after opening	6 months	6 months	6 months	3 months	3 months
14. Batteries	2 (lithium) 3 volts	2 (lithium) 3 volts	2 (lithium) 3 volts	2 (alkaline) AAA	2 (alkaline) AAA 1.5 volts #357
15. Warranty	5 years	5 years	5 years	5 years	6 years
16. Lancing device	Microlet	Microlet	Microlet	Penlet Plus	Penlet Plus

Fast Take®	Precision Q.I.D® MediSense Pen®	Precision Xtra for blood glucose tests (same meter)	Precision Xtra for ketone tests (same meter)	Accusoft® Advantage Complete®	Accusoft® Advantage
LifeScan	MediSense Abbott	MediSense Abbott	MediSense Abbott	Roche Diagnostic	Roche Diagnostic
1.1 to 33.3	1.1 to 33.3	1.1 to 33.3	0 to 6.0	0.5 to 33.3	0.5 to 33.3
15	20	20	30	40	40
150	10	450	450	1000	100
Yes (memory: 150)	Yes (memory: 125)	Yes (memory: 450)	Yes (memory: 450)	Yes Integrated screen (memory: 1000)	Yes (memory: 100)
No	No	No	No	No	No
Automatic calibration	Calibration strip (available from the manufacturer)	Calibration strip (available from the manufacturer)	Calibration strip (available from the manufacturer)	Automatic calibration	CHECK calibration strip
Calibration code on each bottle	Calibration strip in each box	Calibration strip in each box	Calibration strip in each box	Calibration code key in each box	Calibration code key in each box
1.5 µL	3.5 µL	3.5 µL	5 µL	4 µL	4 µL
No	Yes (in the next 30 seconds)	Yes (in the next 30 seconds)	Yes (in the next 30 seconds)	Yes (in the next 15 seconds)	Yes (in the next 15 seconds)
In a bottle (sensitive to humidity)	Packed separately	Packed separately	Packed separately	In a bottle	In a bottle
Yes	Yes	Yes	Yes	Yes	Yes
3 months	18 months (date printed on packet)	18 months (date printed on packet)	18 months (date printed on packet)	18 months (date printed on bottle)	18 months (date printed on bottle)
3 months	3 months	3 months	3 months	3 months	3 months
2 (silver oxide) 1.5 volts #357	Non-replaceable	2 (alkaline) AAA	2 (alkaline) AAA	2 (alkaline) AAA	2 (alkaline) AAA
6 years	For life	4 years	4 years	For life	For life
Penlet Plus	MediSense	MediSense	MediSense	SoftClix Select	SoftClix Select

6. What are the main causes of false readings?

The main causes of erroneous readings are:

1) the capillary glucose meter reader is dirty;

2) the calibration of the capillary glucose meter is wrong;

3) the user forgot to calibrate the meter by omitting to enter the calibration code of the lot of the reactive strips used;

4) the strips have expired;

5) the strips have become humid;

6) the strips have been exposed to extreme temperatures;

7) the drop of blood is too small;

8) wrong technique used;

9) the glucose meter lacks accuracy.

The capillary blood glucose results measured after an overnight fast with the glucose meter should differ by less than 15% from the blood glucose level measured simultaneously in the laboratory.

Example – Fasting, simultaneously:

Result of the capillary blood glucose level: 8.9 mmol/L

Result of the capillary blood glucose level
measured in the laboratory: 10.0 mmol/L

Accuracy of the meter (less than 15% difference)   11%

$$\frac{\text{Capillary blood glucose} - \text{laboratory blood glucose level}}{\text{Laboratory blood glucose level}} \times 100$$

$$\frac{8.9 - 10}{10} \times 100 = \frac{-1.1}{10} \times 100 = 11\%$$

7. How often should people with diabetes measure their capillary blood glucose level?

Usually, people with diabetes are advised to measure their blood glucose level four times a day: **before each meal and before going to bed** (before snacking). Sometimes, the attending physician may also ask you to measure it one to two hours after meals, and more rarely, during the night.

Once the blood glucose level is stabilized, it is possible to reduce these measurements to one, two or three times a day, alternating between different times of the day: before breakfast, before lunch, before dinner or before bedtime.

It is also advisable to measure the capillary blood glucose level every time some discomfort makes you suspect hypoglycemia or hyperglycemia. If you are sick, the blood glucose level should be measured more often.

If some physical activity is performed, it is advisable to measure the blood glucose level before, during and after the activity.

8. How should people with diabetes record this information in their logbook to make analysis easier?

This information should be recorded in your **self-monitoring log-book**. All data of the same nature should be written in a column under a specific heading:

1) capillary blood glucose measurements done **before the breakfast** for the same week should be written in the first column;

2) capillary blood glucose measurements done **after the breakfast** for the same week should be written in the second column;

3) the same should be done for **other capillary blood glucose test measurements** done before and after lunch and dinner, before going to bed (**before snacking**) and during the night;

4) **hypoglycemia** which occurs at times other than the usual four capillary blood glucose measuring periods should be recorded in the next period;

5) a value of **2 mmol/L** should be given to all non-measured blood glucose hypoglycemias;

6) the **weekly average** of these capillary blood glucose tests must be entered at the bottom of each column (the blood glucose level after correction of hypoglycemia should not be used when calculating the mean);

7) **relevant observations** should be noted in the column reserved for this purpose.

Week starting on Sunday: 1 (day) 3 (month) 2001 (year)							
Day of the week	**Capillary blood glucose measurements**						**Comments**
	Breakfast		**Lunch**		**Dinner**		**Bedtime**	
	Before	After	Before	After	Before	After	Before snack	
Sunday	5.2		12.1					
Monday	7.1				8.1			
Tuesday	4.6						4.1	
Wednesday	9.3		10.4			2.3	12.0	
Thursday	5.5				7.2			
Friday	6.8						6.6	
Saturday	3.9		11.3					
AVERAGE	6.1		11.3		7.7		4.3	

The average is calculated by adding up all numbers in the same column and dividing the total by the number of measurements in that column.

Example: $\dfrac{4.1 + 2.3 + 6.6}{3} = \dfrac{13.0}{3} = 4.3$

9. What information should people with diabetes record in their logbook to facilitate better control of their blood glucose?

To facilitate better control of their blood glucose, people with diabetes should record the following information in their logbook:

1) the results and date of the **capillary blood glucose** measurements (in the appropriate columns which correspond to the meals; e.g. "before lunch";

2) the results of measurement of **ketone bodies** in urine or in blood with the date and time (in the "Comments" column);

3) the dosage and name of **each antidiabetic medication** prescribed with the date and time when first taken and at each change of dosage (in the "Comments" column);

4) part of the body where **insulin** was injected, if pertinent (in the "Comments" column);

5) the injection technique, etc. (in the "Comments" column);

6) relevant observations, such as the time of **a hypoglycemic crisis**, presence of infections, etc.

10. Are there other tests besides capillary blood glucose that the doctor could prescribe?

Besides capillary blood glucose, the doctor may prescribe other blood tests to measure fructosamine or glycosylated hemoglobin. These two laboratory analyses reflect the quality of diabetes control:

- for the last two to three weeks in the case of **fructosamine**;

- during the last three months in the case of **glycosylated hemoglobin**.

Notes

Notes

Chapter 5
Measuring ketone bodies in urine

1. What are ketone bodies?

Ketone bodies are the **breakdown products (by-products) of body fats**.

2. What does it mean to have ketone bodies in the urine?

The presence of ketone bodies in urine indicates that the diabetic is using **fat** reserves stored in the body instead of **glucose** due to a **lack of insulin**.

Without insulin, body cells cannot use glucose present in the blood. When this happens, the body receives a message to use energy stored in the form of fat. The breakdown of fats produces **ketone bodies**.

3. Why must people with diabetes check if there are ketone bodies in their urine?

Type 1 people with diabetes must check for ketone bodies in their urine **because their presence means that diabetes is not properly controlled** and there is a risk of ketoacidosis. Ketoacidosis can lead to coma.

4. When must people with diabetes check if there are ketone bodies in their urine?

Usually, people with **type 1 diabetes** should check if they have ketone bodies in the urine. However, the doctor may also recommend these monitoring procedures to **certain people with type 2 diabetes**.

These people should check for the presence of ketone bodies in their urine **when the capillary blood glucose is higher than 15 mmol/L or when requested by their doctor**.

They must continue performing this test, as well as the capillary blood glucose test, four times a day or more if necessary until there are no more **ketone bodies** in their urine and their **capillary blood glucose** is back to **normal**.

They should also perform this test when they have the following symptoms:

1)   **excessive thirst**;

2)   **abdominal pain**;

3)   **excessive tiredness or drowsiness**;

4)   **nausea and vomiting**.

5. What should people with diabetes do when they find ketone bodies in their urine?

People with diabetes who find ketone bodies in their urine should do three things:

1)   **drink a lot** of water to help eliminate the ketone bodies;

2)   **take additional doses of Humulin® R, Novolin® ge Toronto or Humalog® insulin** according to their physician's instructions;

3)   **immediately** call a doctor or go to the emergency room if ketone bodies persist in the urine despite treatment and if the following symptoms appear:

   ▪   abdominal pain;

■ excessive tiredness or drowsiness;

■ nausea and vomiting.

6. How are ketone bodies measured in urine?

Preparing the measuring material

1) Prepare the material: **Ketostix®** test strips, a dry and clean container, and a chronometer.

2) Check the **expiry date** on the test strip container as well as the date the opened container should be thrown out, that is, six months after opening:

   ■ Ketostix® test strips must be stored at room temperature (between 18°C and 25°C)

3) Collect a **fresh** urine sample for testing:

   ■ first, empty your bladder completely and throw out the urine;

   ■ drink one or two glasses of water;

   ■ then urinate into a dry, clean container.

4) Take a test strip from the container and close it **immediately**.

   ■ Compare the color of the test strip with the color chart on the container to make sure that it has not changed, as this could give false results.

Applying the urine sample on the test strip

1) Dip the reactive part of the strip into the fresh urine sample and take it out right away.

2) Let the remaining fluid drip off the test strip onto the edge of the container and start the chronometer.

Reading the results and writing them down

1) **After exactly 15 seconds**, place the test strip near the color chart of the strip vial and compare the result in sufficient light.

2) Write down the result in your self-monitoring logbook.

Negative	Trace	Small	Moderate	Large
-	+	++	+++	++++
0	0.5	1.5	4	8-16 mmol/L

Notes

Notes

Chapter 6

Choosing to eat well

1. What are the objectives of nutrition in the treatment of diabetes?

There are five objectives:

Control of the blood glucose level (blood sugar)

It is mainly **carbohydrates (sugars)** found in food which have an effect on the blood glucose level. Changes in blood glucose can result from an irregular intake of carbohydrates due to **your food choices, the quantities eaten and the distribution of food intake during the day**. To control the blood glucose level, there must be an equilibrium between food intake and insulin produced by the body or received in the form of injections. It should be noted that physical activity and stress also play a role in the control of blood glucose.

Weight control

Carbohydrates, proteins and fats in food and alcohol provide kilocalories (energy). If **the number of kilocalories consumed** is higher than the number of **kilocalories used**, there will be weight gain. People with diabetes who exceed their healthy body weight will usually have more trouble controlling their blood glucose. A **slight weight loss** is often enough to improve the action of insulin and consequently to improve blood glucose control. By being realistic and making progressive changes, your weight loss has a better chance of being permanent.

Control of the lipid (fat) level in blood

Too much fat in the blood can lead to cardiovascular problems.

People with diabetes have a higher risk of developing cardiovascular complications. By following certain rules in the **choice of foods and the amounts consumed**, they may have better control of the level of **triglycerides** and **cholesterol** in their blood. Too much **sugar, fat and alcohol** can increase the level of **triglycerides; too much saturated fats, trans fatty acids** (totally or partially hydrogenated) and **cholesterol** increase the **cholesterol** level.

Meeting your energy, vitamin and mineral needs

From this perspective, the nutrition principles for people with diabetes are not different from those without the condition. They are based on the **Canada's Food Guide to Healthy Eating** which recommends eating **a variety of foods from each group** in quantities that meet your nutritional needs and help you maintain a healthy body weight.

Enjoy eating

Eating is one of life's pleasures. Healthy eating in order to feel well should also be pleasurable. Over the years, we develop eating habits in the context of our familial, social and cultural environments. People with diabetes should learn how to reconcile healthy eating with enjoyable eating and their lifestyle.

2. What should be done to meet these objectives?

To meet these objectives, people with diabetes should have a **healthy meal plan**.

3. What is a healthy meal plan?

A meal plan is a personalized guide indicating the quantities of food to eat in each group, following a precise schedule. It is based on nutritional requirements, medication and other associated diseases. It is essential that people with diabetes meet a dietitian for this purpose.

4. What are the essential characteristics of a meal plan?

The features of a meal plan are quality, quantity, consistency and regularity.

Quality

For quality food intake, you have to make the **best choices**. A meal plan for people with diabetes is usually divided according to food groups. Foods in the same group have similar protein and fat values. These groups are:

- milk

- vegetables

- fruits

- starch

- meat and alternatives

- fats

Foods found in each of these groups are interchangeable for more variety. Each food group is important for **well-balanced meals**.

Quantity

Everyone with diabetes must have a personalized meal plan in which **the number of servings to eat in each group** is indicated according to that person's requirements. **Serving sizes may vary** from one food to another in the same group so that their carbohydrate, protein and fat values are comparable. To become familiar with the sizes of servings, **it is essential, at the beginning, to weigh and measure foods**.

Consistency

For consistency, follow a model menu for the day. We call this the **meal plan**. The meal plan is meant to distribute servings in each food group to be eaten at each of the three meals and snacks. This distribution depends on the type of treatment taken by people with diabetes and the physical activity performed. To achieve consistency in your food intake, you have to follow the model day after day.

Regularity

To achieve regularity, you have to eat your meals and snacks at regular times to avoid discomfort due to hypoglycemia and hyperglycemia.

People with diabetes who are under basal-bolus insulin regimen (i.e. UL*-R**, UL-Humalog®, insulin pump) can be more flexible in the amounts of food they eat and the meal schedule they follow. However, it is not recommended to take breakfast after 9 a.m. Snacks are not compulsory in the morning and afternoon. If you decide to take one, make sure its carbohydrate content is less than 20 g so that you do not have to inject yourself with more insulin. It is recommended that you eat a snack in the evening. This one should be taken as late as possible, that is, after 10 p.m., and it must include carbohydrates.

* _Humulin® U or Novolin® ge Ultralente_
** _Humulin® R or Novolin® ge Toronto_

Notes

Notes

Chapter 7
Carbohydrates: Knowing how to recognize them

1. What are the six food groups?

For a well-balanced diet, a meal plan is usually based on six food groups:

- milk

- vegetables

- fruits

- starch

- meat and alternatives

- fats

Food items in the same group have a similar carbohydrate, protein and fat content.

Among these food groups, it is mostly **those containing CARBOHYDRATES that will have an effect on your blood glucose level.**

2. What are carbohydrates?

The term is used to designate **all types of sugars**: glucose, fructose, lactose, starch, fiber, etc.

3. What is the reference unit for measuring the carbohydrate content of food?

This book uses the teaspoon sugar method:

- 1 teaspoon = 5 g of carbohydrates.

It is based on the method recommended by the American Diabetes Association (ADA), the Quebec Diabetes Association (QDA) and the Quebec College of Dieticians.

To make it easier, all foods containing carbohydrates (except for vegetables) are regrouped so that **one serving provides about 15 g of carbohydrates, equivalent to 3 teaspoons of sugar**. The basic unit is thus 15 g of carbohydrates.

A distinction should be made for people with diabetes using the Canadian Diabetes Association (CDA) system of food choices, because the foods are regrouped differently. **The distinction, for certain food groups, lies in the serving sizes so that the quantity of carbohydrates per serving is not identical**. The following table presents the main differences between the two systems for each serving:

Quantity of carbohydrates per serving		
Food groups containing carbohydrates	Methods recommended by:	
	OPDQ, ADA and QDA	CDA
Milk	12 to 15 g	6 g
Vegetables	0 to 7 g	-
Fruits	15 g	-
Vegetables and fruits	-	10 g
Starch	15 g	15 g
Other carbohydrates	Read the label	10 g

Example: An apple serving		
	Methods recommended by:	
	OPDQ, ADA and QDA	**CDA**
An apple serving is equivalent to:	1 small apple weighing 100 g	½ a medium apple weighing 75 g
Quantity of carbohydrates in a serving of fruits:	15 g	10 g

Consequently, no matter which system is used, it is important to:

1) know how to **recognize the foods** that contain carbohydrates;

2) know the **quantity of carbohydrates in each serving**;

3) **read** the nutrition facts on food product labels;

4) **consult a dietitian** to be informed on the distribution and quantities of carbohydrates to be consumed daily.

4. What are the foods that contain carbohydrates?

Among the six food groups:

Two do not contain or contain minimal carbohydrates:

- **meats and alternatives**

- **fats**

Four contain carbohydrates:

- **milk**

Servings in this group provide **12 to 15 g** of carbohydrates (**2½ to 3 teaspoons of sugar**). The size of the servings varies from one food to another to consistently provide **15 g** of carbohydrates.

Example:	
Foods	1 serving
Milk	250 mL (1 cup)
Plain yogurt	175 mL (¾ cup)

- **vegetables**

Most raw and cooked vegetables contain **minimal carbohydrates**: a **½ cup of vegetables** contains an average of **5 g of carbohydrates or 1 teaspoon of sugar**. Therefore, these food items will be the ones that affect your blood glucose level the least. Their carbohydrate content will count only if you eat large quantities at a time (1½ to 2 cups = 15 g of carbohydrates).

- **fruits**

Servings from this group provide an average of **15 g** of carbohydrates (**3 teaspoons of sugar**). The size of these servings varies from one fruit to another to consistently provide about **15 g** of carbohydrates.

Example:	
Foods	1 serving
Banana	½ small
Grapes	15
Grapefruit juice	½ cup

The carbohydrates in fruit juices with no added sugar are absorbed more rapidly than the carbohydrates in fresh fruits. The dietary fibre of fresh fruits slow the absorption of carbohydrates.

■ **starch**

Servings from this group provide an average of **15 g** of carbohydrates (**3 teaspoons of sugar**). The size of the servings varies from one food to another to consistently provide about **15 g** of carbohydrates.

Example:	
Foods	**1 serving**
Bread	1 slice weighing 30 g
Cooked spaghetti	75 mL (¹⁄₃ cup)
Rusks	2

It is advisable to eat food items rich in dietary fibre, such as whole wheat bread.

5. There are other food items that do not belong to these food groups (e.g. pastries, jams, carbonated soft drinks, etc.). Can they be included in a meal plan?

You do not have to take into account foods that contain **less than 3 g of carbohydrates per serving** (e.g. 2 teaspoons of "light" fruit jams containing 2.5 g of carbohydrates) if you eat **one serving at a time** and if you space the servings throughout the day.

Sugar, honey, jam and **syrup** contain on average **5 g of carbohydrates per 5 mL serving** (1 teaspoon). **One portion at a time** eaten with your meal should have minimum effect on your blood glucose level. Remember that these sugars contain very little vitamins and minerals; they only provide kilocalories.

Pastries, pies, cookies, ice creams, chocolates, chips, crackers, etc. contain **fats** as well as **carbohydrates**. Thus, their energy value (kilo-calories) is high. That is why a person who wishes to lose weight should not eat these food items regularly.

6. How can you find the carbohydrate content of foods that are not in the food groups of the meal plan?

Food value charts can be found in the library (e.g. *Nutrient Value of Some Common Foods*, Health Canada, 1999).

Some fast food restaurants have their own food value charts. Ask them.

The nutrition facts appearing on food product labels is also a good way of knowing the carbohydrate value of foods.

Take crackers, for example:

- useful information on carbohydrate content, either per serving or overall carbohydrate content, is printed in bold letters.

- in this case: 1 serving = 16.8 g = 4 crackers
                                    = 11.4 g of carbohydrates

Note : Do not confuse the weight of a food expressed in grams with its carbohydrate content, which is also expressed in grams.

Nutrition facts
1 serving = 16.8 g (about 4 crackers)

Energy	76 kcal 320 kJ
Protein	1.9 g
Fat	2.5 g
CARBOHYDRATES	**11.4 g**
Sodium	67 mg
Potassium	55 mg

7. How can you include this food item in your meal plan?

If your meal plan is expressed in servings of 15 g of carbohydrates, you have to determine how many crackers will give you 15 g of carbohydrates.

In this case:

- 4 crackers = 11.4 g of carbohydrates

- 5 crackers = 15 g of carbohydrates

If your meal plan is expressed in fixed amounts of carbohydrates per meal, you should find the carbohydrate content according to the number of crackers that you plan to eat.

- 4 crackers = 11.4 g of carbohydrates

- 7 crackers = $\dfrac{11.4 \times 7}{4}$ = 19.95 = 20 g of carbohydrates.

If you are under basal-bolus insulin treatment (i.e. UL*-R**, UL-Humalog®, insulin pump), note the exact carbohydrate value of the serving that you want to eat.

* *Humulin® U or Novolin® ge Ultralente*
** *Humulin® R or Novolin® ge Toronto*

---

8. How much carbohydrates can you eat per day?

The total quantity of carbohydrates that you can eat per day can be determined by your dietitian according to your nutritional needs. This quantity represents, on average, half of your total calorie requirements. Proteins, fats and alcohol provide the remaining calories.

9. Should the same quantity of carbohydrates be eaten every day?

This depends on your treatment:

1) People with diabetes treated with diet only or who have a fixed medical treatment either as oral antidiabetic (hypoglycemic) medications or insulin should eat the same quantity of carbohydrates every day at regular hours.

2) The total amount of carbohydrates have to be spaced out during the day to:

   ■ avoid excessive increases of the blood glucose level after meals for those who are on diet only or those taking oral antidiabetic medications;

   ■ for those treated with insulin, ensure that the intake of carbohydrates coincides with the effect of insulin and physical activity.

> **People who are under basal-bolus insulin treatment (i.e. UL*-R**, UL-Humalog®, insulin pump) can eat quantities of carbohydrates varying from day to day. Meals should always remain balanced without excess fat or protein.**
>
> **Humulin® U or Novolin® ge Ultralente*
> ***Humulin® R or Novolin® ge Toronto*

10. Why are dietary fiber-rich foods preferable?

Foods rich in dietary fiber are strongly recommended because of their beneficial effects on:

1) the **control of blood glucose**, especially after meals;

2)   **constipation**;

3)   **fat levels in blood**;

4)   **appetite**.

Dietary fiber consists of vegetable materials that are **not digested** in the stomach or intestine. Thus, it contains materials that remain in the intestine after foods have been digested.

There are two types of food fiber:

1)   **soluble fiber** found in oats, barley, peas, dried beans, fruits, and vegetables. This fiber helps reduce the cholesterol level and limit the increase of blood glucose after meals.

2)   **insoluble fiber** found in whole wheat and also in peas, dried beans, fruits and vegetables. This fiber facilitates intestinal regularity.

On food product labels, the quantity of fiber is included in the total amount of carbohydrates.

Notes

Chapter 8
Fats: Which fats and how much?

1. Where is fat found?

Some food items contain hidden fats. For example:

- dairy products

- baked goods (croissants, buns, muffins, etc.)

- some breakfast cereals

- fried foods

- fat hidden in meat

- eggs (yolk)

- nuts and almonds

- chips

- chocolate, etc.

Also, there are **fats added** to meals and used during their preparation.

For example:

- butter

- margarine

- oil

- salad dressing

- mayonnaise, etc.

2. Are all fats equal?

Serving for serving, all the following fats are **similar in kilocalories**:

5 mL (1 teaspoon) of:

- butter

- soft margarine

- "light" oil

- meat fat

- fish fat

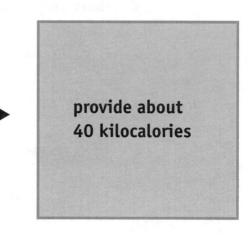

provide about 40 kilocalories

Too much fat often means too many kilocalories.

3. Are fats, proteins and carbohydrates similar in kilocalories?

Weight for weight, fats provide **twice as many kilocalories** as carbohydrates and proteins. In fact:

1 g of fat provides:	9 kilocalories
1 g of protein provides:	4 kilocalories
1 g of carbohydrate provides:	4 kilocalories

4. Which fats are found in food and in the blood?

Five types of fats are found in **FOOD**:

- **saturated fats**

- **trans fatty acids** or **hydrogenated fats**

- **monounsaturated** fats

- **polyunsaturated** fats

- **cholesterol**

Those found mainly in **BLOOD** are:

- **triglycerides**

- **cholesterol** which contains:

  - **HDL-cholesterol**
    (good cholesterol)

  - **LDL-cholesterol**
    (bad cholesterol)

5. What are the main effects of dietary fats on the lipid (fat) levels in blood?*

Fat in foods	Triglycerides	Total cholesterol	HDL-cholesterol	LDL-cholesterol
Excessive fat consumption (more than 30% of energy consumed)	↑	?		
Cholesterol E.g. Giblets (brain, liver, etc.) Egg yolk Cheeses		↑		↑
Saturated fats E.g. Fat in meats, cheeses, etc. Coconut oil Palm oil		↑		↑
Trans fatty acids or hydrogenated fats E.g. Hydrogenated margarine Fried foods Vegetable oil shortening		↑	↓ if consumed in large quantity	↑
Monounsaturated fats E.g. Olive oil, canola oil, etc. Non hydrogenated margarine made from these oils		↓ by replacing saturated fats with mono-unsaturated fats		↓ by replacing saturated fats with mono-unsaturated fats
Polyunsaturated fats E.g. Corn oil, sunflower oil, etc. Non hydrogenated margarine made from these oils Fish (salmon, tuna, etc.) Nuts and grains	↓	↓ by replacing saturated fats with poly-unsaturated fats	↓ if consumed in large quantity	↓ by replacing saturated fats with poly-unsaturated fats

The effects of foods on blood lipids will be observed in individuals predisposed to lipid abnormalities.

? Controversial or needs further study.

In conclusion, it is better to allow a larger proportion of monounsaturated and polyunsaturated fats to prevent an increase in blood lipids.

6. What are the main effects of other factors on the lipid (fat) levels in blood?

Other factors	Triglycerides	Total cholesterol	HDL-cholesterol	LDL-cholesterol
Physical activity	↓	↓	↑	↓
Overweight	↑			
Excessive sugar consumption (60% and more of energy consumption)	↑		↓	
Excessive alcohol consumption	↑			
Cigarette smoking*	↑	↑	↓	↑

The effect of cigarette smoking on blood lipid levels may be related to other associated factors.

7. How to limit fat consumption?

It is important to respect the quantities recommended in your meal plan. However, for **hidden fats**, some advice is given in your meal plan, mainly for meats and alternatives, milk products and starch. You can compare the fat content appearing on the product labeling with that of specific food groups in your meal plan.

Moreover, as far as **added fats** are concerned, you should consult your meal plan to determine the number of fat servings recommended. **A serving of this food group contains 5 g (1 teaspoon) of fat**.

8. Do "light" products contain less fat?

"Light" products do not necessarily contain less fat. *(For more information on this subject, see Chapter 9 – Know how to read food labels: "light," "sugar-free," "fat-free" products, etc.).*

Notes

Chapter 9

Know how to read food labels: "light," "sugar-free," "fat-free" products, etc.

1. What are the types of information found on food product labels?

Three types of information are found on food product labels:
1) **nutritional claims**;
2) **nutrition facts**;
3) **list of ingredients**.

Only the list of ingredients is mandatory.

2. What is a nutritional claim?

A nutritional claim is specific information that the manufacturer has printed on the product label. The terms "light," "sugar-free," "fat-free," etc. are nutritional claims.

When a nutritional claim is made, the manufacturer must provide, somewhere else on the packaging, detailed information on such a claim. This generally appears in the **nutrition facts**.

The following tables give some examples of nutritional claims.

Table 1: Light products

Nutritional claims	Food composition requirements	Comments
Light	Can refer to texture (light oil), taste (light taste) or nutritional value (light in energy, sugar, fat, cholesterol, salt, etc.).	If the term "light" refers to nutritional value (calories, fats, etc.), detailed information must be provided somewhere else on the packaging, either as a decreased percentage compared to the reference food, or in the "Nutrition facts" section. Some light products may have reduced fats, but may contain more carbohydrates than the reference food or the same type of food. Compare the food items carefully.

Table 2: Carbohydrates

Nutritional claims	Food composition requirements	Comments
Carbohydrate-reduced	At least 50% decrease in carbohydrate content compared to the reference food without an increase in energy (calories).	Check the nutrition facts while taking into account the nutritional value given for the serving. Check the fat content.
Low-sugar	≤2 g of carbohydrates per serving.	Check the content in carbohydrates and adapt it to the meal plan.
No sugar added Unsweet-ened	No sucrose or sugar added (e.g. honey, molasses, juices, fructose, glucose).	May contain natural food sugars. Consult the nutrition facts while taking into account the nutritional value given for the serving. Check fat content. Check the carbohydrate content and adapt it to the meal plan.
Sugar-free No sugar Sweet without sugar	At most 1 calorie per 100 g or 100 mL.	

≤ indicates "less than or equal to".

Table 3: Fats

Nutritional claims	Food composition requirements	Comments
Fat-free Contains no fat	$\leq$0.5 g of fat per reference quantity or per serving indicated.	May contain carbohydrates and protein and, thus, calories. Check the nutrition facts while taking into account the nutritional value given per serving.
Low-fat Low in fat	$\leq$ 3 g of fat per serving. $\leq$ 15 g of fat per 100 g of dry matter.	Take into account the nutritional value given per serving.
Reduced in fat	Compared to the reference food, it must have: • at least 25% less fat; • at least 1.5 g less fat per serving; • no increase in energy content.	May contain more carbohydrates than the reference food. May contain a higher proportion of saturated fats.
Light	Food should meet the definitions of composition of the above-mentioned claims.	

$\leq$ *indicates "less than or equal to".*

Table 4: Cholesterol

Nutritional claims	Food composition requirements	Comments
Cholesterol-free Free of cholesterol No cholesterol	≤3 mg of cholesterol per 100 g; ≤2 g of saturated fat per serving; and ≤15% of calories in the form of saturated fatty acids.	Not to be confused with fat content: Foods in this category are low in saturated fat, but overall may contain a lot of fat and/or sugar and, thus, calories. Check the nutrition facts while taking into account the nutritional value given per serving.
Low-cholesterol Low in cholesterol	≤20 mg of cholesterol per 100 g and per serving; and ≤15% of calories in the form of saturated fatty acids.	

≤ indicates "less than or equal to".

Table 5: Calories

Nutritional claims	Food composition requirements	Comments
Calorie-reduced	At least 50% less kilocalories compared to the reference food.	The reduction in calories may be due to either a decrease in fats or in carbohydrates. Check the nutrition facts while taking into account the nutritional value given per serving.
Low-calorie Low in energy Light in calories Light in energy	At least 50% less kilocalories compared to the reference food AND should not contain more than 15 kilocalories per serving.	Eat 1 serving at a time and respect the size of the serving indicated in the nutrition facts. Not more than 2 servings per day.
Calorie-free	≤ 1 kilocalorie per 100 g of food.	

< indicates "less than", or equal to.

3. What is a sugar substitute?

A sugar substitute is a substance that replaces table sugar (sucrose); it gives a sweet taste to foods. Some sugar substitutes, such as aspartame, are calorie-free, while others, such as fructose, contain as many calories as table sugar.

4. What are the sugar substitutes?

The following table lists the sugar substitutes with their daily recommended doses and their characteristics.

Nutritive sweeteners	Acceptable quantity if diabetes is well-controlled	Comments
Fructose	≤3 g/serving	May increase the level of triglycerides and cholesterol if eaten in large quantity. May cause diarrhea if consumption exceeds 50 g/day.
Mannitol*	≤20 g/day	Digestive tolerance evaluated to be 10 to 20 g/day.
Sorbitol*	5 g/serving	A 10-g dose may cause gastrointestinal discomfort.
Xylitol*	≤40 g/day	
Isomalt* Lactitol*	≤50 g/day	Consumption exceeding 50 g/day may cause diarrhea.
Maltitol*	833 mg/kg	
*Sugar-alcohol	≤ indicates "less than or equal to".	

Non nutritive sweeteners	Acceptable daily intake*	Comments
Acesulfame K	15 mg/kg or 1 g/day	Stable under heat. Often combined with other sweeteners.
Aspartame (e.g. Egual®)	40 mg/kg or 2.8 g/day	Unstable under heat: cannot be used for cooking.
Cyclamates (e.g. Sweet'n'Low®)	10 mg/kg or 0.7 g/day	
Saccharine (e.g. Hermesetas®)	< 5 mg/kg or < 0.35 g/day	Low cancer risk observed in rats.
Sucralose (e.g. Splenda®)	9 mg/kg or 0.63 g/day	May be used for cooking.

* For someone weighing 70 kg.
< indicates "less than".

Notes

Notes

Chapter 10
Preparing a menu

1. What are the steps to follow when preparing a menu?

Example of spaghetti with meat sauce

Step 1:

- Refer to your **meal plan**

- Find the number of servings for each group in your sample menu for the appropriate meal.

Example:	
Sample menu	
Lunch	
Milk	1 serving
Vegetables	2 servings
Fruits	1 serving
Starch	**3 servings**
Meats and alternatives	**3 servings**
Fat	3 servings

Step 2:

- Assign the **food items chosen** to the **food group** in which they belong.

Spaghetti with meat sauce

- **Spaghetti = the starch group**

- **Meat sauce = meat and alternatives group**

Step 3:

- Find the **size of a serving** of the specific food in the appropriate group.

Starch group 1 serving = 15 g of carbohydrates		Meat and alternatives	
Food: Spaghetti (cooked)	1 serving: 75 mL (1/3 cup)	Food: Lean ground beef	1 serving: 30 g (1 ounce)

Step 4:

- Decide on the number of servings to be eaten.

Example:

75 mL (1/3 cup) of spaghetti thus:	= 1 serving
250 mL (1 cup)	= 3 servings
Meat sauce containing 90 g (3 ounces)	= 3 servings of meat and alternatives

1) **In this case, all starch servings as well as meat and alternatives servings are used up**. You then have to complete the lunch menu for the other food groups (milk, vegetables, fruits, fats).

2) If your meal plan is divided into fixed amounts of carbohydrate per meal, you should count the carbohydrate content of your spaghetti meal. Complete your menu to obtain the recommended amount of carbohydrates.

If you are under basal-bolus insulin regimen (e.g. UL*-R**, UL-Humalog®, insulin pump), note the carbohydrate value of the serving that you plan to eat (i.e. 1 cup of spaghetti = 45 g of carbohydrates). To assess the amount of food at a glance, you have to practise measuring and weighing that food several times.

*Humulin® U or Novolin® ge Ultralente **Humulin® R or Novolin® ge Toronto.

2. How can you know the nutritional value of a recipe?

To know the nutritional value of a recipe, the following should be indicated:

1) the number of servings* or units that the recipe will give;

2) the nutritional value of a serving or a unit of the recipe in grams (g) of carbohydrate, protein and fat.

Example: Prune muffins

Ingredients: Flour, prunes, sugar, oil, eggs, baking soda
Number of servings: 18 muffins
Nutritional value per muffin: 28 g carbohydrate, 3 g protein, 5 g fat.

---

* *It is important to note that a serving of the recipe does not necessarily correspond to a serving of a food group (i.e. 1 muffin = 1 serving of the recipe and 2 servings each of 15 g of carbohydrates).*

3. How can the nutritional value of a recipe be adapted to your meal plan?

1) If your meal plan is divided into servings of 15 g of carbohydrates, you should determine how many servings of 15 g of food you can obtain (a muffin, in the above-mentioned example), that is:

    28 g ÷ 15 g = 1.9 = 2 portions of 15 g.

2) Know your meal plan well in order to identify what groups the food items will belong to.

3) In the present example, the prune muffin may be counted as one serving of fruit containing 15 g of carbohydrates and one serving of starch containing 15 g of carbohydrates.

4) As far as the nutritional value of protein and fat is concerned, refer to the starch group in your meal plan. The food items in this group contain very little protein and fat. A serving containing 5 g of fat will require adjustment of the meal plan for the group.

5) Adapt the number of servings to the appropriate meal in your sample menu.

Example: Sample menu

Breakfast

Milk	1 serving
Fruits	1 serving
Starch	2 servings
Meats and alternatives	1 serving
Fat	2 servings

In our example, one muffin counts as one serving of fruits, one serving of starch and one serving of fat. You will have to complete your meal with one serving of milk, an additional serving of starch, one serving of meat and alternatives, and one serving of fat.

If the meal plan is divided into fixed amounts of carbohydrates per meal, take note of the carbohydrate content of one or more muffins that you eat. Complete the menu to obtain the recommended amount of carbohydrates.

If you are under basal-bolus insulin regimen (e.g. UL*-R, UL**-Humalog®, insulin pump), take note of the real carbohydrate content of the serving that you plan to eat, that is: One muffin = 28 g of carbohydrates.

*Humulin® U or Novolin® ge Ultralente **Humulin® R or Novolin® ge Toronto.

---

4. How can you know the carbohydrate content of a recipe if you do not know either the number of servings it gives or the nutritional value?

If you do not know the nutritional value of a recipe, you can calculate it from the list of ingredients used in a food composition table. Divide the total values obtained by the number of servings of your recipe.

Notes

Chapter 11
Special situations

A. EATING OUT IN RESTAURANTS

What should be considered when ordering food in a restaurant?

To make up a menu, it is important to **know well your meal plan**. The more familiar you are with your meal plan and serving sizes, the easier it will be to maintain your healthy eating habits in a restaurant.

Do not hesitate to check the composition of foods on the menu. You may telephone the restaurant in advance to know what is on the menu.

Start by making your choice of carbohydrate-containing foods. Choose a simple meal (e.g. grilled meat, starch, vegetables) rather than a dish that contains a combination of foods (e.g. a casserole *au gratin*). This will make it easier to adapt the menu to the food groups in your meal plan.

To avoid excess calories, **pay special attention to fat**. Restaurants often serve foods that contain high levels of fat.

Here are some ways to control the amount of fat in your meals:

- meat, fish:

    - choose a cooking method with no fat (grilled, brochette, or poached in the case of fish);

    - BBQ chicken: leave the skin in your plate.

■ fats (gravy, butter, margarine, salad dressing, cream, etc.):

☐ choose according to the recommended amounts in your meal plan;

☐ ask that gravy and salad dressing be served on the side;

☐ share your French fries with the person who is accompanying you or avoid taking any other fat with your meal.

> To estimate the amount of a serving at a glance, practise measuring and weighing food servings. In some cases, it is after trial and error that you will be able to estimate the carbohydrate content of the meal you choose. You can also compare the carbohydrate content of those food items with the known carbohydrate content of similar frozen commercial foods, for example.

B. DELAYED MEALS

What is the effect of a delayed meal on your blood glucose level?

A meal delayed one hour and more may lead to **hypoglycemia** if you **take oral antidiabetic medications such as sulfonylurea or glinide type**, or if you are **injecting yourself with fixed doses of insulin**.

If the meal is delayed one hour, take a snack containing 15 g of carbohydrates at your usual meal time, and **subtract this serving of carbohydrates from your meal**.

If the meal is delayed two to three hours, take one or two servings of starch with cheese, and **subtract these servings of starch from your meal, or switch the snack in your sample menu with the delayed meal**. If you are taking oral antidiabetic medications or fixed doses of premeal insulin, take them with your delayed meal.

C. ALCOHOL

1. What is the effect of alcohol on your blood glucose level?

Alcoholic beverages that contain sugar can raise your blood glucose level:

- beer, aperitif wines, liqueur and sweet wines.

Alcoholic beverages that do not contain sugar do not raise the blood glucose level if taken in small amounts:

- dry wine and distilled alcohol (gin, rye, rum, whiskey, vodka, cognac, armagnac, etc.).

Drinking alcohol on an empty stomach can cause **hypoglycemia**, especially if you take oral antidiabetic medications such as sulfonylurea or glinide type, or if you are injecting yourself with insulin. All liquor consumption can lead to late hypoglycemia; drinking alcohol with your dinner can cause hypoglycemia during the night. Make sure you have your snack before going to bed. It is sometimes recommended to check your blood glucose level during the night.

2. What factors should be considered when drinking alcohol?

Alcohol has a high energy (calorie) value. Large or frequent consumption may hinder weight loss. Alcohol cannot be put in any food group of your meal plan: it is an extra. Alcohol may increase the level of triglycerides (lipids in the blood).

Do not drink alcohol if your diabetes is not well-controlled.

Alcohol should never be taken on an empty stomach.

In the general population, **women** should not take more than one drink a day, and **men** no more than two drinks a day. One drink is equivalent to:

■ 1½ ounces (45 mL) of distilled alcohol

■ 4 ounces (125 mL) of dry wine

■ 2 ounces (60 mL) of dry sherry

■ 12 ounces (375 mL) of beer

> **Remember that just one drink of alcohol can lead to hypoglycemia. Alcohol should be consumed slowly. A single drink is sufficient to cause alcohol breath. The symptoms of hypoglycemia and alcohol intoxication being quite similar, people around you may confuse one for the other and delay appropriate treatment. Do not drink alcohol before, during or after physical exercise. Wear a bracelet or pendant that identifies you as a person with diabetes to avoid any confusion between alcohol intoxication and a hypoglycemic reaction.**

D. SICK DAY ACTION PLAN

1. What are the effects of minor illnesses on diabetes?

Minor illnesses, such as a cold, the flu or gastroenteritis, can impair diabetes control. The disease is a stress for the body. The blood glucose level will tend to increase for two reasons:

1) there is an increase in hormones that stimulates the glucose stored in the liver to enter the bloodstream;

2) these same hormones will also increase the resistance of cells to insulin and thus decrease the entry of glucose into the cells.

2. What precautions should be taken when a minor illness occurs?

In case of a minor illness, such as a cold or the flu, medical consultation is generally unnecessary. **Five important rules** should be followed:

1) Continue to take your oral antidiabetic medications and/or insulin doses; it is possible that your insulin needs will increase. If you are being treated with insulin, ask your doctor to create an insulin adjustment scale according to your capillary blood glucose measurements.

Example:
Adjustment of insulin doses during sick days

2 units of Regular, Toronto or Humalog® insulin for each 2 mmol/L above 14 mmol/L before each meal and when going to bed.

---

2) **Measure your capillary blood glucose (blood sugar level)** at least **four times a day or every two hours if high values are observed**.

3) **Check if ketone bodies are present in your urine if your blood glucose level is higher than 15 mmol/L.**

4) **Drink a lot of water** to avoid dehydration.

5) Take the **amount of carbohydrates recommended with meals and snacks in the form of easily digested foods**.

3. Should the same be done in case of gastroenteritis?

Gastroenteritis usually causes **diarrhea** and sometimes **vomiting**, which can lead to **dehydration** and loss of **electrolytes** (sodium and potassium).

To allow you to continue taking the quantity of carbohydrates recommended in your meal plan, a three-phase approach is recommended to guide you in the choice of foods to avoid dehydration and treat the diarrhea and vomiting.

Phase 1: Liquid food

1) Stop eating solid foods. Avoid milk and milk-based drinks.

2) Drink water, broth or *consommé* (clear broth) at any time without any restriction.

3) Drink 250 mL (1 cup) of the following preparation every hour:

Preparation of 1 liter or 4 cups:

- 500 mL (2 cups) of water

- 500 mL (2 cups) of sugar-free orange juice

- 5 mL (1 teaspoon) of salt

250 mL (1 cup) of this drink provides about 15 g of carbohydrates.

---

4) Try to take the amount of carbohydrates recommended per day.

5) Progressively replace the drink by other sugar-free fruit juices (except for prune juice), flavored gelatine (Jell-O®), caffeine-free, decarbonated soft drinks.

Phase 2: Foods low in fiber

1) Gradually add foods containing **15 g of carbohydrates** to complete the total amount of carbohydrates recommended in your meal plan at meals and snack times.

   Fruit group:

   ■ 1 raw, grated apple

   ■ ½ ripe banana

   ■ 125 mL (½ cup) of sugar-free orange juice

   Starch group:

   ■ 2 rusks

   ■ 8 soda crackers

   ■ 4 Melba® toasts

   ■ 1 slice of toasted bread

   ■ 75 mL (⅓ cup) of plain pasta

   ■ 75 mL (⅓ cup) of rice

2) Add cooked vegetables: carrots, beets, asparagus, yellow or green beans.

3) Add lean meats (white chicken or turkey meat), fish cooked without fat or mild cheese.

Phase 3: Return to normal food

Progressively resume your normal intake of food according to your meal plan for persons with diabetes, while avoiding:

1) **foods which can give gas**:

   - corn

   - legumes (chick peas, red beans, etc.)

   - cabbage

   - onion

   - garlic

   - raw vegetables

2) **foods which may be irritating**:

   - fried foods

   - spices

   - chocolate

   - coffee

   - cola

> **IMPORTANT! Notify your doctor or go to emergency if one of the following occurs:**
> - **your capillary blood glucose level is higher than 20 mmol/L;**
> - **you have a medium to high level of ketone bodies in your urine;**
> - **you vomit continuously and are unable to drink;**
> - **your temperature is higher than 38.5°C for more than 48 hours.**

E. TRAVELLING

1. Planning a trip?

When preparing for a trip, always consider the following factors:

1) make sure that your diabetes is **well-controlled** (see your doctor),

2) obtain a **letter from your doctor** testifying that you have diabetes and describing your treatment, especially if your condition requires insulin injections;

3) carry **identification** showing that you are a person with diabetes;

4) find out what costs are covered by **insurance** companies for pre-existing diseases that involve medical expenses abroad and for returning home in case of medical emergency;

5) be familiar with the **habits and customs** of the country you are visiting;

6) **inform the transportation company** that you are a person with diabetes.

2. What are the precautions that you should take when carrying material and medications necessary for the treatment of diabetes?

Keep in your handbag (and not in your stored luggage) all that you need for treating your diabetes, that is:

1) twice the amount of insulin required in case of breakage or if it is not available abroad;

2) a thermal pack to protect your insulin;

3) a self-monitoring kit;

4) medication to control diarrhea and vomiting as well as antibiotics;

5) extra food in case of hypoglycemia or a delayed meal.

3. Are there special recommendations to follow during a trip?

During the trip, you are recommended to:

1) **closely follow your usual schedule of meals and snacks**, especially if you are under split-mixed insulin regimen (NPH with rapid-acting or short-acting) *(see Chapter 14 – Insulins)*;

2) continue to **check your capillary blood glucose level regularly** to verify that your diabetes is always well-controlled since there is a risk of changing your habits;

3) **always** keep **extra food** on hand.

4. When treating diabetes with the "split-mixed" insulin regimen, how should the insulin doses be adjusted during a trip involving a time zone change of more than three hours?

The "Split-mixed" insulin regimen is a combination of **intermediate** (Humulin® N or Novolin® ge NPH) and **short-acting** insulin (Humulin® R or Novolin® ge Toronto) or **rapid-acting** insulin (Humalog®) which is injected before breakfast and dinner.

Take, for example, a Montreal-Paris trip, where the time zone difference is six hours. Suppose you are taking the following insulin doses:

- NPH 16 units and short-acting 8 units before your breakfast

- NPH 6 units and short-acting 6 units before your dinner

Departure:

Montreal-Paris. The day of departure being shorter by six hours, **reduce NPH by 50% before your dinner and divide your short-acting insulin in two**.

Meal	Capillary blood glucose	Insulin	Meal
Montreal: breakfast	yes	NPH 16 units, S.A.* 8 units	normal
Montreal: lunch	yes	———	normal
Montreal: dinner	yes	NPH 3 units, S.A.* 3 units	50%
During flight: dinner	yes	S.A.* 3 units	50%
During flight: breakfast	yes	S.A.* 8 units	normal

*   *S.A.: Short-acting. (Humulin® R or Novolin® ge Toronto).*

Return:

Paris-Montreal. On the return trip, the day is longer by six hours. **Eat an additional meal** (that is, 50% of your usual dinner), preceded by an **additional short-acting insulin** dose equaling 50% of your usual short-acting dose.

Meal	Capillary blood glucose	Insulin	Meal
Paris: breakfast	yes	NPH 16 units, S.A.* 8 units	normal
Paris: lunch	yes	————	normal
During flight: dinner	yes	NPH 6 units, S.A.* 6 units	normal
Montreal: dinner	yes	S.A.* 3 units	50%

* S.A.: *Short-acting. (Humulin® R or Novolin® ge Toronto).*

5. When treating diabetes with the "prandial-bedtime" insulin regimen, how should the insulin doses be adjusted during a trip involving a time zone change of more than three hours?

The "Prandial-bedtime" insulin regimen consists of a **short-acting** insulin injection (Humulin® R or Novolin® ge Toronto) or **rapid-acting** insulin (Humalog®) before each meal and an injection of intermediate-acting insulin (Humulin® N or Novolin® ge NPH) at bedtime.

Take, for example, a Montreal-Paris trip, where the time zone difference is six hours. Let's suppose you usually take:

- Short-acting 8 units before your breakfast

- Short-acting 8 units before your lunch

- Short-acting 8 units before your dinner

- NPH 8 units before bedtime

Departure:

Montreal-Paris. The day of departure is shorter by six hours. **Advance the time of the NPH dose and reduce it by 50% while dividing the short-acting insulin dose in two**.

Meal	Capillary blood glucose	Insulin	Meal
Montreal: breakfast	yes	S.A.* 8 units	normal
Montreal: lunch	yes	S.A.* 8 units	normal
Montreal: dinner	yes	NPH 4 units, S.A.* 4 units	50%
During flight: dinner	yes	S.A.* 4 units	50%
During flight: breakfast	yes	S.A.* 8 units	normal

*   S.A.: Short-acting. (Humulin® R or Novolin® ge Toronto).

Return:

Paris-Montreal. On the return trip, the day is longer by six hours. **Eat an additional meal** (50% of your usual dinner), **preceded by 50% of your usual short-acting insulin injection before dinner**.

Meal	Capillary blood glucose	Insulin	Meal
Paris: breakfast	yes	S.A.* 8 units	normal
Paris: lunch	yes	S.A.* 8 units	normal
During flight: dinner	yes	S.A.* 8 units	normal
Montreal: dinner	yes	S.A.* 4 units	50%
Montreal: snack at bedtime	yes	NPH 8 units	snack

*   S.A.: Short-acting. (Humulin® R or Novolin® ge Toronto).

6. When treating diabetes with the "basal-bolus" insulin regimen, how should the insulin doses be adjusted during a trip involving a time zone difference of more than three hours?

The "basal-bolus" insulin regimen consists of one injection of **short-acting** insulin (Humulin® R or Novolin® ge Toronto) or **rapid-acting** insulin (Humalog®) before each meal and one injection of long-acting insulin

(Humulin® U or Novolin® ge Ultralente) at bedtime. The premeal insulin is usually given according to the amount of carbohydrates to be ingested.

Take, for example, a Montreal-Paris trip, where the time zone difference is six hours. Let's suppose you usually take:

- UL 12 units at bedtime

- Short-acting 1.2 unit/10 g of carbohydrates before your breakfast

- Short-acting 1.0 unit/10 g of carbohydrates before your lunch

- Short-acting 1.0 unit/10 g of carbohydrates before your dinner

Because of the long-lasting action of UL insulin, it is not necessary to change the dose.

Departure:

Montreal-Paris. The day of departure is shorter by six hours. **Take the UL dose** before your departure. While you may wait to take your dinner in the plane, **you are advised to eat a light meal before leaving**.

Meal	Capillary blood glucose	Insulin	Meal
Montreal: breakfast	yes	S.A.* 1.2 units per 10 g of carbohydrates	normal
Montreal: lunch	yes	S.A.* 1 unit per 10 g of carbohydrates	normal
Montreal: dinner	yes	UL 12 units, S.A.* 1 unit per 10 g of carbohydrates	50%
During flight: dinner	yes	S.A.* 1 unit per 10 g of carbohydrates	normal or 50%
During flight: breakfast	yes	S.A.* 1.2 units per 10 g of carbohydrates	normal

*   S.A.: Short-acting. (Humulin® R or Novolin® ge Toronto).

Return:

Paris-Montreal. On the return trip, the day is longer by six hours. **Eat an additional meal (about 50% of a normal meal)** in the evening with your usual short-acting dose before your meal.

Meal	Capillary blood glucose	Insulin	Meal
Paris: breakfast	yes	S.A.* 1.2 units per 10 g of carbohydrates	normal
Paris: lunch	yes	S.A.* 1 unit per 10 g of carbohydrates	normal
During flight: dinner	yes	S.A.* 1 unit per 10 g of carbohydrates	normal
Montreal: dinner	yes	S.A.* 1 unit per 10 g of carbohydrates	normal or 50%
Montreal: snack at bedtime	yes	UL 12 units	snack

*   *S.A.: Short-acting. (Humulin® R or Novolin® ge Toronto).*

7. When treating diabetes with the "premixed" insulin regimen, how should the insulin doses be adjusted during a trip involving a time zone difference of more than three hours?

The "premixed" insulin regimen consists of a mixture of **intermediate and short-acting** insulin injection (Humulin® 30/70, Humulin® 50/50, Novolin® ge 30/70, Novolin® ge 50/50, etc.) or a mixture of intermediate and rapid-acting insulin (Humalog Mix-25®) before breakfast and dinner.

Take, for example, a Montreal-Paris trip, where the time zone difference is six hours. Let's suppose you are taking Humulin 30/70:

■   20 units before your breakfast

■   10 units before your dinner

Departure:

Montreal-Paris. The departure day is shorter by six hours. **Take half of your dinner insulin dose before dinner** and the other half in flight, during the meal.

Meal	Capillary blood glucose	Insulin	Meal
Montreal: breakfast	yes	Humulin 30/70 20 units	normal
Montreal: lunch	yes	——	normal
Montreal: dinner	yes	Humulin 30/70 5 units	50%
During flight: dinner	yes	Humulin 30/70 5 units	50%
During flight: breakfast	yes	Humulin 30/70 20 units	normal

Return:

Paris-Montreal. On the return trip, the day is longer by six hours. **Take an additional dinner** (50% of your usual dinner), **preceded by an insulin dose equivalent to 50% of your usual dose taken before your meal**.

Meal	Capillary blood glucose	Insulin	Meal
Paris: breakfast	yes	Humulin 30/70 20 units	normal
Paris: lunch	yes	——	normal
During flight: dinner	yes	Humulin 30/70 10 units	normal
Montreal: dinner	yes	Humulin 30/70 5 units	50%
Montreal: snack at bedtime	yes	——	snack

Notes

Notes

Chapter 12
Oral antidiabetic medications

1. What is an oral antidiabetic medication?

An oral antidiabetic medication is a medication you **take orally to lower your blood glucose level**.

2. How many classes of oral antidiabetic medications are there?

There are five classes of oral antidiabetic medications:

Class	Medications
Sulfonylureas	Chlorpropamide (e.q. Diabinese®)
	Gliclazide (e.g. Diamicron®)
	Glyburide (e.g. Diaßeta®, Euglucon®)
	Tolbutamide (e.g. Apo-Tolbutamide®)
Meglitinides	Repaglinide (e.g. GlucoNorm®)
Biguanides	Metformin (e.g. Glucophage®)
Thiazolidinediones	Pioglitazone (e.g. Actos®)
	Rosiglitazone (e.g. Avandia®)
Alpha-glucosidase inhibitors	Acarbose (e.g. Prandase®)

3. When should you take oral antidiabetic medications for the treatment of diabetes?

Oral antidiabetic medications are taken for the treatment of type 2 diabetes, **if diet, exercise and weight loss are not sufficient to normalize the blood glucose level**.

REMEMBER! Oral antidiabetic medications do not replace, but rather complement, diet, exercise and weight loss.

---

4. What are the main characteristics of sulfonylureas (e.g. glyburide, gliclazide)?

1) **Mechanism of action:** They **stimulate the release of insulin from the pancreas**. They are ineffective if insulin-producing pancreatic cells are not functioning.

2) **Adverse effects: Hypoglycemia** is the principal adverse effect associated with the sulfonylureas. It may appear at any time of the day or night. The dosage should therefore be adjusted. To minimize the risks of hypoglycemia, meals and snacks should be eaten at fixed times according to the meal plan. You are advised not to take these medications at bedtime.

3) **Best time to take them:** It is advisable to take sulfonylureas **before meals, but never more than 30 minutes before**.

5. What are the main characteristics of meglitinides (e.g. repaglinide)?

1) **Mechanism of action:** Just like the sulfonylureas, they **stimulate the release of insulin from the pancreas**. They are therefore ineffective if the insulin-producing pancreatic cells are not functioning. Meglitinides are different from the sul-

fonylureas in that their **action is faster and of shorter duration**.

2) **Adverse effects: Hypoglycemia** is an adverse effect that can occur with the meglitinides. Their dosage should therefore be adjusted. To minimize the risks of hypoglycemia, meals and snacks should be eaten at fixed times according to the meal plan. It is not advisable to take these medications at bedtime.

3) **Best time to take them:** It is advisable to take the meglitinides **before meals, but never more than 15 minutes before**.

6. What are the main characteristics of the biguanides (e.g. metformin)?

1) **Mechanism of action:** They mainly reduce the production of glucose by the liver.

2) **Adverse effects: Gastrointestinal problems, especially diarrhea**, are adverse effects most often attributed to the biguanides. They sometimes leave a metallic taste in the mouth. If they are taken alone, the biguanides rarely cause hypoglycemia.

3) **Best time to take them:** It is advisable to take the biguanides **at mealtime** to minimize adverse gastrointestinal effects.

7. What are the main characteristics of the thiazolidinediones (e.g. pioglitazone, rosiglitazone)?

1) **Mechanism of action:** They **reduce resistance to insulin**. In other words, they make insulin more effective. This increases the use of glucose, especially by the muscles, but also by adipose (fat) tissues.

2) **Adverse effects: Edema (swelling due to water retention)** and weight gain are possible adverse effects. If they are taken alone, the thiazolidinediones rarely cause hypoglycemia.

3) **Best time to take them:** It is advisable to take the thiazolidinediones at the same time every day. It is not necessary to take them with meals.

8. What are the main characteristics of the alpha-glucosidase inhibitors (e.g. acarbose)?

1) **Mechanism of action:** They **delay the absorption of carbohydrates ingested with meals**. Therefore, the increase of blood glucose after meals is reduced.

2) **Adverse effects: Gastrointestinal problems**, especially **bloating and flatulence (gas)**, are the principal adverse effects attributed to alpha-glucosidase inhibitors. If they are taken alone, alpha-glucosidase inhibitors do not cause hypoglycemia.

3) **Best time to take them:** To be effective, it is **compulsory** to take alpha-glucosidase inhibitors **after the first bite of food**.

Main mechanisms of action of oral antidiabetic medications

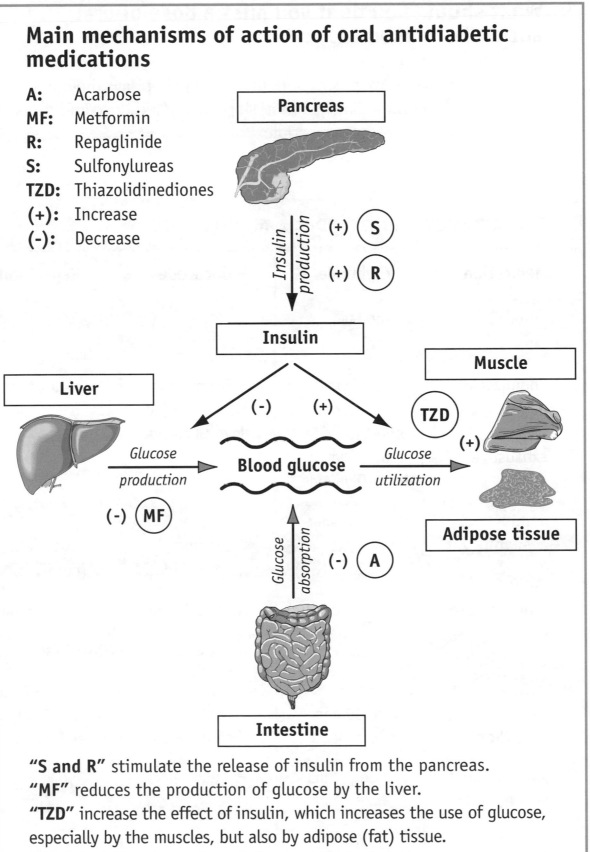

A: Acarbose
MF: Metformin
R: Repaglinide
S: Sulfonylureas
TZD: Thiazolidinediones
(+): Increase
(-): Decrease

Pancreas

Insulin production

(+) S

(+) R

Insulin

Liver

Muscle

(-)   (+)

TZD

Glucose production

Blood glucose

Glucose utilization

(+)

(-) MF

Adipose tissue

Glucose absorption

(-) A

Intestine

"S and R" stimulate the release of insulin from the pancreas.
"MF" reduces the production of glucose by the liver.
"TZD" increase the effect of insulin, which increases the use of glucose, especially by the muscles, but also by adipose (fat) tissue.
"A" delays the absorption of dietary carbohydrates.

9. What should you do if you miss a dose of oral antidiabetic medication?

1) If you remember soon after the appropriate time, take the dose immediately. If not, skip the missed dose and go back to your regular schedule.

The main oral antidiabetic medications

Medication	Glyburide	Gliclazide	Repaglinide
Class	Sulfonylurea	Sulfonylurea	Meglitinide
Commercial name (list not exhaustive)	Diaßeta Euglucon Apo-Glyburide Gen-Glybe Novo-Glyburide	Diamicron Gen-Gliclazide Novo-Gliclazide	GlucoNorm
Commercial availability	2.5 and 5 mg tablets (divisible in two)	80 mg tablets (divisible in four)	0.5, 1 and 2 mg tablets (not divisible)
Daily dosage	1.25 to 20 mg	40 to 320 mg	1 to 16 mg
Number of daily doses	1 to 3	1 to 3	2 to 4 (according to the number of meals)
Best time to take them	0 to 30 min before meals	0 to 30 min before meals	0 to 15 min before meals
Most frequent adverse effects	Hypoglycemia	Hypoglycemia	Hypoglycemia
Risk of hypoglycemia	Yes	Yes	Yes

2) **Do not double dose**.

3) It is advisable not to take sulfonylureas or meglitinides at bedtime, as this increases the risk of hypoglycemia.

4) **Alpha-glucosidase inhibitors** are effective only if they are taken **with the meal**. If you forget, it is useless to take them after the meal.

Acarbose	Metformin	Pioglitazone	Rosiglitazone
Alpha-glucosidase inhibitor	Biguanide	Thiazolidinedione	Thiazolidinedione
Prandase	Glucophage Apo-Metformin Gen-Metformin Novo-Metformin	Actos	Avandia
50 and 100 mg tablets (divisible in two)	500 mg (divisible in two) and 850 mg (not divisible) tablets	15, 30 and 45 mg tablets (not divisible)	2, 4 and 8 mg tablets (not divisible)
50 to 300 mg	250 to 2500 mg	15 to 45 mg	4 to 8 mg
1 to 3	1 to 4	1	1 to 2
With meals	With meals	With or without food	With or without food
Flatulence, bloating, diarrhea	Diarrhea, metallic taste	Edema, weight gain	Edema, weight gain
No	No	No	No

Notes

Chapter 13
Non-prescription drugs

1. Are non-prescription drugs free of side effects?

No medication is totally free of side effects. Sometimes, non-prescription drugs can have harmful side effects. It is, therefore, important to follow instructions carefully.

2. How do you choose non-prescription drugs considering your health condition?

Some non-prescription drugs must be avoided or used with caution in certain illnesses or if taken at the same time as prescription medications. You are strongly advised to **consult your pharmacist** when choosing a non-prescription drug.

3. How can your pharmacist help you?

When describing your symptoms to your pharmacist, he/she may suggest an appropriate non-prescription drug for your condition. In some cases, he/she will recommend that you avoid taking the non-prescription drug as it may be harmful or ineffective in your case. He/she may also recommend some simple non-pharmacologic ways (e.g. staying in bed, drinking lots of water, etc.). Finally, it is possible that the pharmacist will ask you to consult your doctor if he/she feels that your condition requires it.

It is advisable that you have all your prescriptions filled at the same pharmacy. This will allow the pharmacist to give you the best advice.

4. What types of non-prescription drugs should be avoided or used with caution by people with diabetes?

1) **oral decongestants** (against nasal congestion);

2) medications containing **sugar**;

3) **keratolytic** preparations (for the treatment of corns, calluses and warts);

4) high doses of **acetylsalicylic acid** (e.g. Aspirin® or ASA).

5. Why must oral decongestants be used with caution?

Oral decongestants (e.g. Sudafed®) are medications (syrups, tablets, powder packs) that reduce nasal congestion. Most oral decongestants contain an ingredient known as "sympathomimetic" (e.g. pseudo-ephedrine) that can have a **hyperglycemic** effect, especially if the recommended doses are exceeded. Overconsumption of this type of product is frequent, as cold remedies often contain a mixture of ingredients (e.g. against cough, fever, etc.), and people often take two different products in which the common ingredient is a sympath-omimetic decongestant. Thus, they often take twice the dose without knowing it.

This type of oral decongestant is likewise not recommended if you have vascular problems, hypertension, hyperthyroidism and cardiac diseases, such as angina.

As alternative treatments, you are advised to drink a lot of water, keep the ambient air well humidified and use a saline nasal vaporizer.

If the congestion persists, you can try a nasal vaporizer decongestant but for no more than 72 hours.

6. Why should non-prescription drugs containing sugar be used with caution?

It is important for people with diabetes to know which medications contain sugar to avoid losing control of their blood glucose level. All medications containing **20 kilocalories and more per dose or which provide 80 kilocalories and more per day** should be avoided, or taken into account in your meal plan. The sugar content is usually printed on the packaging. Sugar is an ingredient found not only in syrups, but also in powder packs, chewable tablets, lozenges, etc.

There are many "sucrose-free" preparations. These usually contain sugar substitutes. They can be used by people with diabetes, at the recommended dose, except if the active ingredient is contra-indicated for another reason.

7. Why should keratolytic skin preparations (for the treatment of corns, calluses and warts) be used with caution?

Adhesive plasters, disks, ointments and gels containing products such as salicylic or tannic acid are often used for the treatment of corns, calluses and warts. These acids are **very irritating**. Consult a doctor, a podiatrist or a nurse specialized in foot care before using such products.

8. Why should high doses of acetylsalicylic acid be used with caution?

High doses of acetylsalicylic acid (e.g. Aspirin®, Anacin®, Entrophen®, etc.) can cause **hypoglycemia**. This effect can be produced if the daily dose exceeds 3000 mg, which is equal to more than nine tablets of 325 mg per day or six tablets of 500 mg per day.

Acetaminophen (e.g. Tylenol®, Atasol®, etc.) does not contain acetylsalicylic acid and is a safe alternative in case of fever and pain.

9. Should "natural" products be taken by people with diabetes?

"Natural" products are not free from potential adverse effects. You are strongly advised to seek the advice of your pharmacist before taking such products. He/she will check for possible interactions with your other medications and for contraindications, depending on your health condition.

The composition of these products is not always known and can vary from one lot to another. Inform your doctor about the natural products that you are taking.

If you decide to take a natural product, pay particular attention to your capillary blood glucose level. Some products may increase or lower your blood glucose level (e.g. glucosamine may elevate blood glucose).

10. At the pharmacy, is there a simple way of knowing which non-prescription drugs should be used with caution or avoided?

In the Province of Quebec, the "Ordre des pharmaciens du Québec" has developed a program known as the "Drug Caution Code." The Code consists of six letters, each corresponding to a specific caution. These code letters usually appear on price stickers or on the pharmacy shelf where the medication is found.

The **code letter "E"** is specifically addressed to **people with diabetes**. Indeed, all products bearing "code E" are **not recommended**. "Code E" identifies three types of products:

  1) oral decongestants;

  2) medications with sugar equivalent to 20 kilocalories and more per dose or 80 kilocalories and more per day;

3) keratolytic preparations (for the treatment of corns, calluses and warts).

A personalized "Drug Caution Code" card filled out by your pharmacist will indicate the code letters which apply to you.

If you are not a Quebec resident, check with your pharmacist to find out if there is a similar "Drug Caution Code" program in your area.

Notes

Chapter 14
Insulins

1. How does insulin lower the blood glucose level?

The main role of insulin is to allow glucose in the bloodstream to enter the cells of the body. Its transport into the cells lowers the blood glucose level.

2. When is insulin used for the treatment of diabetes?

Insulin is systematically used for the treatment of **type 1 diabetes** because, in this case, the pancreas does not produce any insulin. It is also used for the treatment of **type 2 diabetes** if diet, exercise, weight loss and oral antidiabetic medications **are not enough to control blood glucose**.

3. How are insulins produced?

Insulins are mainly manufactured in the laboratory according to bio-genetic techniques using bacteria or yeast genetically programmed to produce insulin.

There are two categories of insulin:

1) **Human insulin:** This insulin is identical to insulin produced by the human pancreas. All insulins called Humulin® or Novolin® fall into this category.

2) **Analogue insulin:** This insulin is similar to insulin produced by the human pancreas. However, its structure has been slightly changed in relation to human insulin in order to give it new properties. Humalog® and Humalog® Mix 25 are some examples of this type of insulin.

Some types of insulin may also be of animal origin (purified pork insulin). These insulins are rarely ever used. They are mentioned here only for information purposes.

4. What are the different types of insulin?

Insulins can be classified according to their **time of action**. There are six types:

1) **rapid-acting** insulin

2) **short-acting** insulin

3) **intermediate-acting** insulin

4) **long-acting** insulin

5) **premixed** insulin made of a mixture of **rapid-acting** and **intermediate-acting** insulins

6) **premixed** insulin made of a mixture of **short-acting** and **intermediate-acting** insulins.

5. What are the action times of the different insulin types?

Type of insulin	Onset of action after injection	Peak action after injection	Duration of action after injection
Rapid-acting Humalog®	0 to 15 minutes	1 to 2 hours	3 to 4 hours
Short-acting Humulin® R (Regular) Novolin® ge Toronto	30 minutes	2 to 4 hours	6 to 8 hours
Intermediate-acting Humulin® N Novolin® ge NPH Humulin® L Novolin® ge Lente	1 to 2 hours	6 to 12 hours	18 to 24 hours
Long-acting Humulin® U Novolin® ge Ultralente	4 to 5 hours	8 to 20 hours (small or no peak of action)	24 to 28 hours
Premixed rapid-acting and intermediate-acting Humalog® Mix 25*	0 to 15 minutes	1 to 2 hours and 6 to 12 hours	18 to 24 hours

Type of insulin	Onset of action after injection	Peak action after injection	Duration of action after injection
Premixed short-acting and intermediate-acting** Humulin® 10/90*** Novolin® ge 10/90 Humulin® 20/80 Novolin® ge 20/80 Humulin® 30/70 Novolin® ge 30/70 Humulin® 40/60*** Novolin® ge 40/60 Humulin® 50/50*** Novolin® ge 50/50	30 minutes	2 to 4 hours and 6 to 12 hours	18 to 24 hours

*   *Humalog® Mix 25 is a mixture of 25% lispro insulin (rapid-acting insulin) and 75% lispro protamine insulin (intermediate-acting insulin).*

**   *The first number corresponds to the percentage of short-acting insulin in the mixture, and the second number corresponds to the percentage of intermediate-acting insulin of the NPH type in the mixture.*

*** *These preparations will be gradually removed from the market by the manufacturer.*

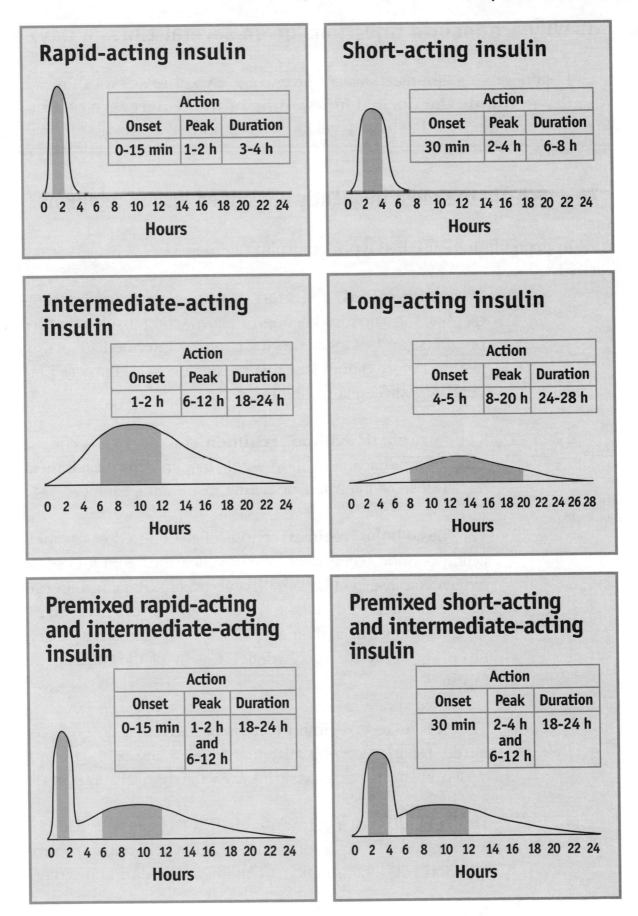

Rapid-acting insulin

Action		
Onset	Peak	Duration
0-15 min	1-2 h	3-4 h

Hours

Short-acting insulin

Action		
Onset	Peak	Duration
30 min	2-4 h	6-8 h

Hours

Intermediate-acting insulin

Action		
Onset	Peak	Duration
1-2 h	6-12 h	18-24 h

Hours

Long-acting insulin

Action		
Onset	Peak	Duration
4-5 h	8-20 h	24-28 h

Hours

Premixed rapid-acting and intermediate-acting insulin

Action		
Onset	Peak	Duration
0-15 min	1-2 h and 6-12 h	18-24 h

Hours

Premixed short-acting and intermediate-acting insulin

Action		
Onset	Peak	Duration
30 min	2-4 h and 6-12 h	18-24 h

Hours

6. Why are insulin injections given several times a day?

In general, insulin injections are given one, two, three or four times a day **to mimic the normal functioning of the pancreas** in order to maintain the blood glucose level as close to normal as possible.

7. Which are the most frequently prescribed insulin regimens?

In general, there are five types of insulin regimens:

1) The **"split-mixed" regimen** consists of injecting intermediate-acting and rapid-acting or short-acting insulins before breakfast and dinner. The injection of intermediate-acting insulin before dinner is sometimes given at bedtime to prevent hypoglycemia during the night.

2) The **"prandial-bedtime" regimen** consists of injecting a dose of rapid-acting or short-acting insulin before each meal and a dose of intermediate-acting insulin at bedtime.

3) The **"basal-bolus" regimen** consists of injecting a dose of rapid-acting or short-acting insulin before each meal and a dose of long-acting insulin at bedtime (basal insulin). Basal insulin can also be administered in the form of multiple injections of intermediate-acting insulin during the day. Premeal insulins are often given according to carbohydrate content of the meal to be ingested.

4) The **"Premixed" regimen** consists of injecting a dose of premixed insulin made of a mixture of rapid-acting or short-acting insulin and intermediate-acting insulin before breakfast and dinner.

5) The **"Combined" regimen** consists of injecting a dose of intermediate-acting or long-acting insulin at bedtime in combination with oral antidiabetic medications during the day.

8. At what times should insulin injections be given?

Before **meals**:

1) **Rapid-acting insulin** must be injected **just before meals** (or **not more than 15 minutes before**), whether it is pre-mixed or not. This allows the peak action of insulin to coincide with the peak absorption of carbohydrates ingested;

2) **Short-acting insulin** must be injected **15 to 30 minutes before meals**, whether it is premixed or not. This allows the peak action of insulin to coincide with the peak absorption of carbohydrates ingested;

3) **Intermediate-acting insulin** in the "split-mixed" regimen is given **before meals** as with the rapid-acting or short-acting insulins. Sometimes, the injection of intermediate-acting insulin before dinner must be delayed until bedtime to prevent hypoglycemia during the night.

Before **bedtime**:

1) **Intermediate-acting or long-acting insulin** given as basal insulin is often injected at about **10 p.m.** Treatment must be given as much as possible at a fixed time. This permits the peak of action (if any) to coincide with breakfast.

9. What is the most common adverse effect of insulin treatment?

Hypoglycemia is the most common adverse effect seen in people treated with insulin. The risk of hypoglycemia is much higher during the peak action of insulin.

10. How is it possible to maintain good control of diabetes with insulin injections?

To control diabetes well with insulin injections, it is important to **apply self-discipline** and respect certain rules:

1) closely follow your **meal plan**;

2) **measure your capillary blood glucose level regularly**;

3) **adjust your insulin doses yourself**, after obtaining the necessary training from your diabetes care team.

11. At what time of the day should people with diabetes treated with insulin measure their capillary blood glucose?

If your diabetes is being treated with insulin, measure your blood glucose **before meals and at bedtime (before your snack)**. Sometimes, it is helpful to measure blood glucose after the meal (one to two hours after the first mouthful, especially when using rapid-acting insulin) or even during the night (at about 2 a.m.). You are also advised to measure your capillary blood glucose level each time you feel discomfort which seems related to hypoglycemia or hyperglycemia.

Notes

Notes

Chapter 15

Preparation and injection of one type of insulin

1. What types of insulin injectors are available?

There are two types of insulin injectors:

1) **The syringe type.** A syringe has a reservoir, a plunger and a fine needle. It can have different capacities, either of 100 units, 50 units or 30 units. The finer the needle, the greater the gauge. For example, a 30 gauge needle is finer than a 29 gauge needle. However, the finer the needle, the shorter the length (8 mm in contrast to 12.7 mm).

2) **The pen-injector.** This device is slightly larger than a pen and is made up of three parts: a cap which covers a fine needle, the cartridge holder which contains the insulin cartridge, and the pen body which includes a plunger. A dosage button allows you to choose the desired dose.

2. How do you prepare the injection of one type of insulin with a syringe?

There are three steps in the preparation and injection of one type of insulin.

Preparing the materials

1) **Wash your hands** with soap and dry well.

2) **Lay out** the syringe with needle, the bottle of insulin, an alcohol swab and a cotton ball.

3) Check the bottle label to make sure you are using the right **type of insulin**.

4) Check **both expiry dates** on the label: the date recorded by the manufacturer and the date you recorded when you opened the bottle.

   ■ After opening, a bottle of insulin can be used for **one month** if kept at room temperature (between 18°C and 25°C). Keeping the insulin at room temperature reduces pain at the injection site.

   ■ You should always keep **a spare bottle** of insulin in the refrigerator (at a temperature between 2°C and 10°C).

   ■ It is recommended to use **a 29 gauge syringe of 12.7 mm** to inject Humulin® U or Novolin® ge Ultralente. This makes it easier to inject and avoids blocking the needle.

Preparing the insulin

1) If the insulin is **opaque**, roll the bottle between your hands to mix the suspension well. **Do not shake it**.

2) **Disinfect the cap of the bottle** with the alcohol swab.

3) **Pull back the plunger** of the syringe to draw in air up to the marking of the dose to be injected.

4) **Insert the needle** into the rubber cap of the insulin bottle.

5) **Inject the drawn in air** into the bottle.

6) **Turn over the bottle and the syringe** until they are upside down.

7) **Gradually pull back the plunger** until it reaches the required dose.

   ■ Make sure there are no air bubbles in the syringe to avoid injecting an insufficient amount of insulin.

   ■ Push the plunger until all air bubbles disappear.

   ■ Check the syringe. If any insulin has been lost, repeat Step 6.

Injecting insulin and recording the data

1) **Choose the injection site.**

   ■ Do not inject insulin into a limb or part of your body that you will be using for a physical activity (your leg, for example, if you're going to take a walk – or your arm, if you're going to play tennis, etc.).

2) In **choosing the injection site**, take into account the condition of the skin.

   ■ Do not inject into skin that has a depression, bump or growth or that is bruised, red or painful.

3) **Disinfect the injection site** with an alcohol swab and let it dry.

4) **Pinch the skin** between your thumb and index finger, and hold it like that until you finish injecting.

5) Hold the syringe like a pencil and **stick the needle into your skin at a 90-degree angle**.

   ■ The insulin must be injected subcutaneously (into the tissue beneath the skin). Injecting at a 90-degree angle allows most people to reach the required depth. However, **a thin person** can inject at a **45-degree angle** to make sure that the insulin penetrates into the subcutaneous tissue, not into the muscle beneath it.

6) **Inject the full amount of insulin** by pushing the plunger as far as it will go.

- **Do not pull the plunger back.** You can injure the skin if you raise the plunger to check if you got the right spot.

7) **Withdraw the needle** and press down gently on the injection site with the cotton ball.

- Blood at the injection site may indicate that you have penetrated a muscle. If so, starting with your next injection, it is recommended to inject insulin at a 45-degree angle.

- The presence of a white zone around the site may indicate that you have not injected deeply enough.

8) Each time the dosage is changed, **record the number of units** and type of insulin injected in the appropriate column of your logbook.

3. What are the different types of pen-injectors available?

There are several models of pen-injectors (*list revised as of February 1, 2001*):

Pen-injector	Manufacturer	Cartridge	Graduation	Dosage dial
B-D Mini Pen	Becton/ Dickinson	1.5 mL	0.5 unit at a time	0.5 to 15 units
B-D Pen 1.5 mL	Becton/ Dickinson	1.5 mL	1 unit at a time	1 to 30 units
B-D Pen 3.0 mL	Becton/ Dickinson	3.0 mL	2 units at a time	2 to 60 units
Pre-loaded disposable injector	Eli Lilly	3.0 mL	1 unit at a time	1 to 60 units
Humulin N Pen				
Humalog Pen				
Humalog Mix 25 Pen				
Huma Pen Ergo	Eli Lilly	3.0 mL	1 unit at a time	1 to 60 units
Novolin-Pen 1.5 mL	Novo Nordisk Canada Inc.	1.5 mL	1 unit at a time	1 to 40 units
Novolin-Pen 3.0 mL	Novo Nordisk Canada Inc.	3.0 mL	1 unit at a time	1 to 70 units
Pre-loaded disposable injector	Novo Nordisk Canada Inc.	3.0 mL	2 units at a time	2 to 78 units
Novolin Set: Toronto, 30/70, NPH				

To find out what type of insulin and needles can be used with a particular pen-injector, check the product monograph.
If you use two types of insulin which are not premixed, you can use two pen-injectors.

4. How do you prepare for insulin injection using a pen-injector?

The preparation and injection of insulin with a pen-injector are done in three steps:

Preparing the materials

1) **Wash your hands** with soap and dry well.

2) **Lay out** the pen-injector with its insulin cartridge and needle, an alcohol swab, and a cotton ball.

3) Check the **type of insulin** and the amount remaining in the cartridge.

4) Check both **expiry dates** on the label: the date recorded by the manufacturer and the date you recorded when you opened the bottle.

  - A cartridge in use should be kept for no longer than a month if stored at room temperature (between 18°C and 25°C).

  - Maximum storage temperatures for cartridges are 25°C for Humulin®, 30°C for Humalog® and 37°C for Novolin®.

  - Cartridges not in use must be kept in the refrigerator, at a temperature between 2°C and 10°C, until the expiry date recorded by the manufacturer.

  - Do not refrigerate the pen-injector so as not to damage it and to avoid forming air bubbles in the cartridge.

Selecting the insulin dosage

1) **Bring opaque insulin to a uniform appearance.** Turn the opaque insulin cartridge over and back ten times or more. The glass marble inside the cartridge will move from one end to the other.

2) **Fill the empty space in the needle** by injecting one unit of insulin at a time, until you see a drop of insulin at the tip of the needle when pointed upwards.

3) **Choose the insulin dose** by turning the dosage button until it reaches the required number of units.

Injecting the insulin and recording the data

1) **Choose the injection site.**

   ■ Do not inject insulin into a limb or part of your body that you will be using for a physical activity (your leg, for example, if you're going to take a walk – or your arm, if you're going to play tennis, etc.).

   ■ **Choose the injection site** in the selected area by taking into account the condition of the skin.

   ■ Don't inject into skin that has a depression, bump, bruise, is red or painful.

2) **Disinfect the skin well** with an alcohol swab and let it dry.

3) **Pinch the skin between your thumb and index finger**, then hold it there until you finish injecting with a needle 8 to 12 mm long.

4) It is recommended that you do not pinch the skin when using shorter needles (**5 or 6 mm**).

5) Hold the pen-injector like a pencil and **stick the needle into your skin at a 90-degree angle**.

- The insulin must be injected subcutaneously (into the tissue beneath the skin). Injection at a 90-degree angle allows most people to reach the correct depth. However, a **thin person** can inject at a **45-degree angle** to make sure that the insulin penetrates into the subcutaneous tissue, and not the muscle beneath. This is not necessary when using shorter needles (5 or 6 mm).

6) **Inject the full amount of insulin** by pushing the plunger as far as it will go.

- Leave the needle in place for about **15 seconds**.

7) **Remove the needle** and press down gently on the injection site with the cotton ball.

- Blood at the injection site may indicate that you have penetrated a muscle. If so, starting with your next injection, it is recommended to inject insulin at a 45-degree angle or use short needles (**5 or 6 mm**).

- The presence of a white area around the injection site may indicate that you have not injected deeply enough.

- Remove the needle from the cartridge as soon as the injection is completed.

- Use a fresh needle each time you inject.

8) Each time the dosage is changed, **record the number of units** and the type of insulin injected in the appropriate column of your personal logbook.

Notes

Notes

Chapter 16

Preparation and injection of two types of insulin

1. What precautions must be taken when mixing two types of insulin in the same syringe?

When you have to mix clear and opaque insulin in the same syringe, you must take two precautions:

1) Intermediate-acting insulin (Humulin® N or Novolin® ge NPH) must be loaded before clear, short-acting insulin (Humulin® R or Novolin® ge Toronto) or clear, rapid-acting insulin (Humalog®). **Opaque insulin is easily detected if injected by accident into a bottle of clear insulin.**

    ■   The correct sequence to follow in mixing insulins in the same syringe is a controversial subject. The most important concern is to avoid any contamination of one insulin by the other.

    ■   In general, it is not advisable to mix long-acting (Humulin® or Ultralente) or intermediate-acting insulin (Humulin® L or Novolin® ge Lente) in the same syringe with short-acting (Humulin® R or Novolin® ge Toronto) or rapid-acting insulin (Humalog®).

2) If a drop of opaque insulin is accidentally injected into a bottle of clear insulin, you must **throw out the contaminated bottle** as it will not have its usual peak and duration of action. The contaminated insulin may cause poor glycemic control.

2. How do you prepare an injection of two types of insulin?

Preparing the materials

1) **Wash your hands** with soap and dry well.

2) **Lay out** the syringe with needle, the insulin bottles, an alcohol swab and a cotton ball.

3) Check both bottle labels to make sure you have the **correct types of insulin**.

4) Check **both expiry dates** on the labels: the dates recorded by the manufacturers and the dates you recorded when you opened the bottles.

   ■ Once opened, a bottle of insulin should not be used for more than **one month** if kept at room temperature (between 18°C and 25°C). Keeping the insulin at room temperature reduces pain at the injection site.

   ■ You should always keep **a spare bottle of insulin** in the refrigerator (at a temperature between 2°C and 10°C).

   ■ It is recommended to use a **29 gauge syringe of 12.7 mm** to inject Humulin® U or Novolin® ge Ultralente: this makes it easier to inject and avoids blocking the needle.

Loading the insulin

1) **Roll the container** of opaque insulin between your hands to properly mix the insulin in suspension. **Do not shake it.**

2) **Disinfect the cap** of the opaque and clear insulin bottles well with the alcohol swab.

3) **Inject air** into the clear insulin bottle.

   ■ Pull back the plunger of the syringe. Draw in air up to the number of units of clear insulin to be injected. Insert the needle into the rubber cap of the clear insulin bottle and inject the air into the bottle. Do not touch the insulin or load it into the syringe. Remove the needle from the bottle.

4) **Inject air** into the opaque insulin bottle.

   ■ Pull back the plunger on the syringe. Draw in air up to the number of units of opaque insulin to be injected. Insert the needle into the rubber cap of the opaque insulin bottle and inject the air into the bottle. Leave the needle in the bottle.

5) **Load the required dose** of opaque insulin.

   ■ Hold the opaque insulin bottle and the syringe upside down. Slowly pull the plunger back to draw the required number of units of opaque insulin into the syringe. Remove the needle from the bottle.

   ■ Make sure there are no air bubbles in the syringe. Otherwise, you risk injecting an insufficient amount of insulin.

   ■ Push the plunger until all air bubbles disappear.

   ■ Check the syringe to make sure you have not lost any insulin. If any insulin has been lost, repeat the previous step.

6) **Load the required dose** of clear insulin.

   ■ Turn the clear insulin bottle upside down and insert the needle into the rubber cap. Make sure no opaque insulin escapes into the clear insulin container. Slowly pull the plunger back to draw the required number of units of clear insulin into the syringe. Remove the needle from the bottle.

If too much clear insulin is loaded

- **Throw out** the insulin loaded in the syringe.

- **Start** the process from the beginning.

If opaque insulin gets into the clear insulin bottle

- **Throw out** the clear insulin bottle.

- **Start over** the process from the beginning with a new bottle.

Injecting the insulin and recording the data

1) **Choose the injection site**

   - Do not inject insulin into a limb or part of your body that you will be using for a physical activity (your leg, for example, if you're going to take a walk – or your arm, if you're going to play tennis, etc.).

2) **Choose the injection site** in the selected area, taking into account the condition of the skin.

   - Do not inject into skin that has a depression, bump, bruise, is swollen, red or painful.

3) **Disinfect the skin** with an alcohol swab and let it dry.

4) **Pinch the skin** around the injection site between your thumb and index finger, and hold it like that till the injection is completed.

5) Hold the syringe like a pencil and **stick the needle into your skin at a 90-degree angle**.

   ■ The insulin must be injected subcutaneously (into the tissue beneath the skin). Injection at a 90-degree angle allows most people to reach the required depth. However, **a thin person** can inject at a **45-degree angle** to make sure that the insulin penetrates into the subcutaneous tissues, and not into the muscle.

6) **Inject the full amount of insulin** by pushing the plunger as far as it will go.

   ■ Do not pull the plunger back. You can injure the skin if you raise the plunger to check if you got the right spot.

7) **Remove the needle** and press down gently on the injection site with the cotton ball.

   ■ Blood at the injection site may indicate that you have penetrated a muscle. If so, starting with your next injection, it is recommended to inject insulin at a 45-degree angle.

   ■ The presence of a white area around the injection site may indicate that you have not injected deeply enough.

8) Each time the dosage is changed, **record the number of units** and type of insulin injected in the appropriate column of your personal logbook.

Notes

Chapter 17
Injection of insulin:
Rotation of injection sites

1. Where are the main areas of the body where insulin may be injected?

Insulin may be injected in eight different areas of the body, known as **"injection areas"**:

Areas 1 and 2	**ABDOMEN:**	left and right sides, almost everywhere, except for 1 cm (½ inch) around the belly button
Areas 3 and 4	**ARMS:**	the anterior-external parts
Areas 5 and 6	**THIGHS:**	the anterior-external parts
Areas 7 and 8	**BUTTOCKS:**	the fleshy parts

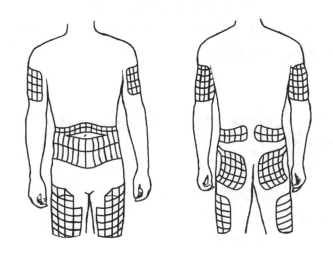

2. How many injection sites are there in each area?

In each **injection area**, there are many zones where insulin may be injected; these are called **"injection sites"**. You can make use of the entire surface within each injection area, but do not use **the same injection site more than once a month**.

3. What is the distance between each injection site of the same injection area?

Each **injection site** must be at least 1 cm (½ inch) from the site of the previous injection.

Injection sites:

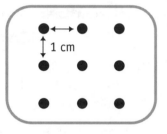

4. Why must the injection site be changed for each insulin injection?

You must change the **injection site for each insulin injection** to prevent **lipodystrophy**: bumps and cracks from repeated injections at the same site. Besides being unattractive, damage to subcutaneous tissue interferes with insulin absorption and may cause problems in the control of your blood glucose.

5. Does the injection area influence the absorption of insulin injected?

Yes. For the same insulin, the speed of absorption varies according to the injection area used.

Listed below is the relative speed of absorption by region, from the most rapid to the slowest:

A: Abdomen

B: Arms

C: Thighs

D: Buttocks

6. What other factors influence the rate of insulin absorption?

Intense exercise increases the rate of absorption if the insulin has been injected into a part of the body being exercised.

- For example, insulin injected into a thigh will be absorbed more quickly if you take a walk or play tennis after the injection.

Other factors, such as heat (sun, bath, shower, etc.), depth of the injection, massage near the injection site, may affect the rate of absorption.

> **A pregnant woman should not inject insulin into her abdomen unless she can fold the skin (between her fingers). Otherwise, she could damage the skin.**

7. How can you ensure that the quantity of insulin in the blood varies as little as possible in relation to the site used for injection?

To ensure that the quantity of **insulin** present in the blood varies as little as possible relative to the site used for injection, you may do the following:

1) Inject short-acting or rapid-acting insulin into the **abdomen** – either alone or mixed with intermediate-acting insulin. Change the injection site each time.

2) For greater convenience, before your lunch, you can regularly use your arm as an injection area for short-acting or rapid-acting insulin. This will ensure that the peak effect of the midday injection will be the same every day, allowing you to adjust the dosage accordingly.

3) Use the **thighs or buttocks** for injecting intermediate-acting or long-acting insulin that is not mixed with short-acting or rapid-acting insulin. This will ensure that absorption is as slow as possible.

4) If you inject yourself at different times of the day, use the same injection area every day at a particular time.

5) Each injection area is associated with a certain absorption rate. Choose a particular area based on how fast the specific insulin acts and the activity level of that particular time of day.

For example:

Thighs:	slow absorption rate
Ultralente Insulin:	long-acting rate
Bedtime:	reduced activity

To summarize:

Type of insulin	Area of the body where insulin is injected		
	Abdomen	Arm	Thighs and buttocks
Short-acting or rapid-acting alone	Area of choice	Before the midday meal for most convenience	——
Short-acting or rapid-acting and intermediate-acting mixed	Area of choice	——	——
Intermediate-acting alone	——	——	Area of choice
Long-acting alone	——	——	Area of choice

Notes

Chapter 18
Storage of insulin

1. Where should insulin be stored and for how long?

Insulin vials

1) Once opened, insulin vials may be used for no more than **one month** if stored at room temperature (between 18°C and 25°C). Keeping insulin at room temperature reduces pain at the injection site.

   - Insulin vials in use can tolerate temperatures up to 25°C for such brands as Humulin® and Novolin® and up to 30°C for Humalog®.

   - Never leave insulin exposed to direct sunlight or heat.

   - As soon as you open a vial of insulin, record the date on the label.

2) You should **always** keep a spare vial of each type of insulin in the refrigerator (between 2°C and 10°C) in case of an emergency, such as a broken vial, for example. If properly stored, an unopened vial can be used until the expiry date indicated by the manufacturer.

3) Insulin vials must never be allowed to freeze. Since you can't tell by its appearance whether insulin has undergone freezing, you must throw out any insulin that may have been frozen.

Insulin cartridges

1) Insulin cartridges may be used for no more than **one month** if stored at room temperature (between 18°C and 25°C).

2) Insulin cartridges in use can tolerate temperatures up to 25°C for such brands as Humulin®, 30°C for such brands as Humalog® and 37°C for such brands as Novolin®.

3) You should always keep spare insulin cartridges in the refrigerator (between 2°C and 10°C). If properly stored, an unopened cartridge can be used until the expiry date indicated by the manufacturer.

4) You must not store a pen-injector in the refrigerator. Refrigeration could cause damage or create air bubbles in the cartridge.

5) Insulin cartridges must never be allowed to freeze. Since you can't tell by its appearance whether insulin has undergone freezing, you must throw out any insulin that may have been frozen.

Disposable pen-injectors

1) Disposable pen-injectors may be used for no more than **one month** if stored at room temperature (between 18°C and 25°C).

2) Pen-injectors in use can tolerate temperatures up to 30°C for such brands as Humalog® Pen and Humalog® Mix 25 Pen, and 37°C for such brands as Novolin Set® ge.

3) You should always keep spare disposable pen-injectors in the refrigerator (between 2°C and 10°C). If properly stored, a disposable pen-injector can be used until the expiry date indicated by the manufacturer.

Prefilled insulin syringes

1) Prefilled insulin syringes should be stored in the refrigerator (between 2°C and 10°C).

2) The maximum length of storage time depends on the particular brand. Brands such as Humulin® and Humalog® can be stored for three weeks. Novolin® insulin brands should be stored for the shortest possible time.

3) It is recommended that prefilled insulin syringes be stored in a vertical or diagonal position with the needle (and its cap) pointing upward. This prevents insulin particles from clogging the needle.

2. Why are all these precautions necessary for storing insulin?

All these necessary precautions should be taken since insulin is a fragile protein. It may lose its effectiveness if stored too long or exposed to extreme temperatures, leading to poor control of blood glucose.

3. What appearance should insulin have and when should we throw it out?

1) **Rapid-acting or short-acting insulin**
   (Humalog®, Humulin® R, Novolin® ge Toronto)

   ■ These types of insulin are **clear solutions resembling water**.

   ■ **Throw it out** if:

      ☐ it looks cloudy;

      ☐ it is thick;

    ☐   it contains solid particles;

    ☐   it has been exposed to extreme temperatures (heat or cold).

2) **Intermediate-acting, long-acting or premixed insulin** (e.g. Humulin® N, Novolin® ge NPH, Humulin® L, Novolin® ge Lente, Humulin® U, Novolin® ge Ultralente, Humalog® Mix 25, Humulin® 30/70, Novolin® ge 30/70)

■   These types of insulin **are opaque or milky** and may leave a deposit. Before using, roll the vial between your hands till the content becomes **uniform and homogeneous. Do not shake it.**

■   Long-acting insulin (Humulin® U, Novolin® ge Ultralente) needs to be mixed longer to become uniform and homogeneous.

■   If there is a whitish deposit at the bottom of the vial, **turn it upside down** several times. **Do not shake it.**

■   **Throw it out** if:

    ☐   a deposit remains at the bottom of the vial;

    ☐   specks float in the insulin;

    ☐   particles have collected along the walls of the vial, giving it a frosted appearance;

    ☐   it has been exposed to extreme temperatures (heat or cold).

Notes

Notes

Chapter 19
Adjustment of insulin doses

1. What blood glucose levels should be maintained when adjusting insulin doses?

In general, it is recommended to keep glucose levels as close as possible to normal: **between 4 and 7 mmol/L before meals and at bedtime** (before snack if any) and **between 5 and 11 mmol/L one to two hours after meals**.

2. What are the six golden rules for adjusting insulin doses?

Before trying to adjust your insulin doses, it is important that you take time to analyze your blood glucose levels. Examine and average your last three blood glucose levels for each period of the day (morning, noon, evening and bedtime). Do not go back more than seven days. Consider only levels registered since the last time you adjusted your insulin dosage.

Here are the six golden rules:

1) In your calculations, do not include any measurement that is less than 4 mmol/L or more than 7 mmol/L which is associated with a **situation that is sporadic, exceptional and explainable**.

2) Never adjust your insulin dosage based on **only one blood glucose test**.

3) Always adjust **only one insulin dose** at a time at one period of the day.

4) Begin by correcting **hypoglycemia**, starting with the first hypoglycemia of the day.

- A hypoglycemic situation is present when:

  □ the average level is below 4 mmol/L for a given period of the day;

  or

  □ the average level is over 4 mmol/L for a given period of the day, but there have been three non-consecutive hypoglycemic readings in the last seven days or the last two readings have been hypoglycemic.

- Assign a value of 2 mmol/L to any hypoglycemia that has not been measured.

- A hypoglycemic reading taken outside the four periods of the day when blood glucose is usually measured should be entered for the next period (for example, enter a hypoglycemic reading taken in the afternoon in the "before dinner" column).

5) Afterwards, correct the **hyperglycemic** situation: which is an average of more than 7 mmol/L for a given period of the day. Start with the first period of the day (before breakfast), then the second (before lunch), etc.

6) After changing your insulin dosage, wait at least two days before making any new adjustment. A longer waiting period is required for long-acting insulin.

3. What are the different insulin regimens that are prescribed most frequently?

In general, there are five major insulin regimens:

1) The **"split-mixed" insulin regimen** consists of injecting an intermediate-acting (e.g. Humulin® N, Novolin® ge NPH) and rapid-acting (Humalog®) or short-acting (Humulin® R, Novolin® ge Toronto) insulin before breakfast and dinner. Sometimes, the injection of intermediate-acting insulin before dinner must be delayed until bedtime to prevent hypoglycemia during the night.

2) The **"prandial-bedtime" insulin regimen** consists of injecting one dose of rapid-acting (Humalog®) or short-acting (Humulin® R, Novolin® ge Toronto) insulin before each meal and one dose of intermediate-acting insulin (e.g. Humulin® N, Novolin® ge NPH) before bedtime.

3) The **"basal-bolus" regimen** consists of injecting one dose of long-acting insulin (Humulin® U, Novolin® ge Ultralente) at bedtime (basal insulin) and one dose of rapid-acting (Humalog®) or short-acting (Humulin® R, Novolin® ge Toronto) insulin before each meal. Basal insulin can also be administered in the form of multiple injections of intermediate-acting insulin during the day. Premeal insulins are often given according to carbohydrate content of the meal to be ingested.

4) The **"premixed" regimen** consists of injecting one dose of premixed insulin (e.g. Humulin® 30/70, Novolin® ge 30/70, Novolin® ge 50/50, Humalog® Mix 25) before breakfast and dinner.

5) The **"combined" regimen** consists of injecting one dose of intermediate-acting insulin (e.g. Humulin® N, Novolin® ge NPH) or long-acting insulin (Humulin® U, Novolin® ge

Ultralente) at bedtime in addition to oral antidiabetic medications during the day.

4. In the "split-mixed" regimen, which blood glucose levels are affected by each insulin injected?

Which insulin:	will affect the blood glucose level before:
The intermediate-acting insulin[a] before dinner	→ breakfast
The rapid-acting[b] or short-acting insulin[c] before breakfast	→ lunch
The intermediate-acting insulin[a] before breakfast	→ dinner
The rapid-acting[b] or short-acting insulin[c] before dinner	→ bedtime

[a] Humulin® N, Novolin® ge NPH, Humulin® L, Novolin® ge Lente
[b] Humalog®
[c] Humulin® R, Novolin® ge Toronto

The blood glucose level at any given time always reflects the effect of the **preceding** insulin dose injected.

5. How should insulin doses be adjusted in the "split-mixed" regimen?

In general, in case of **hypoglycemia (blood glucose level below 4 mmol/L)**, as defined in the golden rules, the appropriate insulin dose should be reduced by two units at a time. However, if the total daily dose of insulin is less than or equal to 20 units, reduce the dose by only one unit at a time.

In general, in case of **hyperglycemia (blood glucose level above 7 mmol/L)**, as defined in the golden rules, the appropriate insulin dose should be increased by two units at a time. However, if the total daily dose of insulin is less than or equal to 20 units, increase the dose by only one unit at a time.

After any change of an insulin dose, you must wait at least two days before making any new adjustment. In case of hypoglycemia or hyperglycemia, do not wait more than one week to adjust the appropriate insulin dose.

6. In the "prandial-bedtime" regimen, which blood glucose level is affected by each insulin injected?

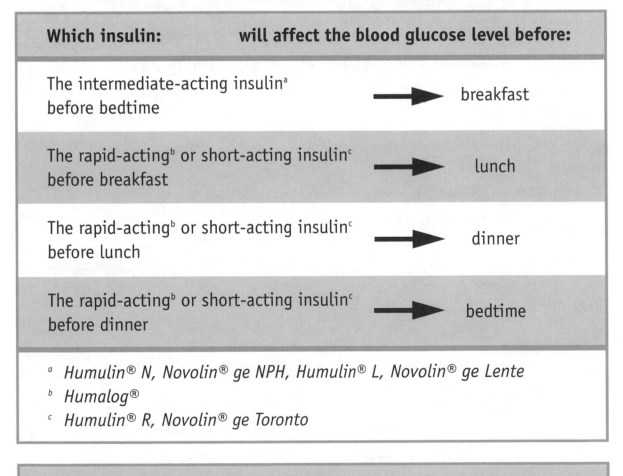

Which insulin:	will affect the blood glucose level before:
The intermediate-acting insulin[a] before bedtime	→ breakfast
The rapid-acting[b] or short-acting insulin[c] before breakfast	→ lunch
The rapid-acting[b] or short-acting insulin[c] before lunch	→ dinner
The rapid-acting[b] or short-acting insulin[c] before dinner	→ bedtime

[a] *Humulin® N, Novolin® ge NPH, Humulin® L, Novolin® ge Lente*
[b] *Humalog®*
[c] *Humulin® R, Novolin® ge Toronto*

The blood glucose level at any given time always reflects the effect of the **preceding** insulin dose injected.

7. How should the insulin doses be adjusted in the "prandial-bedtime" regimen?

In general, in case of **hypoglycemia (blood glucose level below 4 mmol/L)**, as defined in the golden rules, the appropriate insulin dose should be reduced by two units at a time. However, if the total daily dose of insulin is less than or equal to 20 units, **reduce** the dose by only one unit at a time.

In general, in case of **hyperglycemia (blood glucose level above 7 mmol/L)**, as defined in the golden rules, the appropriate insulin dose should be increased by two units at a time. However, if the total daily dose of insulin is less than or equal to 20 units, **increase** the dose by only one unit at a time.

After any change of an insulin dose, you must wait at least two days before making any new adjustment. In case of hypoglycemia or hyperglycemia, do not wait more than one week to adjust the appropriate insulin dose.

8. In the "basal-bolus" regimen, which blood glucose level is affected by each insulin injected?

Which insulin:		will affect the blood glucose level before:
The long-acting insulin[a] at bedtime	➤	breakfast
The rapid-acting[b] or short-acting insulin[c] before breakfast	➤	lunch
The rapid-acting[b] or short-acting insulin[c] before lunch	➤	dinner
The rapid-acting[b] or short-acting insulin[c] before dinner	➤	bedtime

[a]Humulin® U, Novolin® ge Ultralente
[b]Humalog®
[c]Humulin® R, Novolin® ge Toronto

The blood glucose level at any given time always reflects the effect of the **preceding** insulin dose injected.

9. How should insulin doses be adjusted in the "basal-bolus" regimen?

In case of **hypoglycemia (blood glucose level below 4 mmol/L)**, as defined in the golden rules:

1) During the night or before breakfast, the dose of long-acting insulin (Humulin® U, Novolin® ge Ultralente) should be reduced by two units at a time. However, if the total daily dose of long-acting insulin is less than or equal to 10 units, reduce the dose by only one unit at a time.

2) Before lunch and dinner or before bedtime, **reduce** the appropriate dose of insulin (Humulin® R, Novolin® ge Toronto or Humalog®) by 0.2 unit/10 g of carbohydrates (if counting carbohydrates) at a time. However, if the dose of this insulin is less than or equal to 0.5 unit/10 g of carbohydrates, reduce the dose by only 0.1 unit/10 g of carbohydrates at a time.

In case of **hyperglycemia (blood glucose level above 7 mmol/L)**, as defined in the golden rules:

1) During the night or before breakfast, the dose of long-acting insulin (Humulin® U, Novolin® ge Ultralente) should be increased by two units at a time. However, if the total daily dose of long-acting insulin is equal to or less than 10 units, **increase** the dose by only one unit at a time.

2) Before lunch and dinner or before bedtime, **increase** the dose of insulin (Humulin® R, Novolin® ge Toronto or Humalog®) by 0.2 unit/10 g of carbohydrates (if counting carbohydrates) at a time. However, if the dose of this insulin is less than or equal to 0.5 unit/10 g of carbohydrates, **increase** the dose by only 0.1 unit/10 g of carbohydrates at a time.

After any change of a dose of Humulin® R, or Novolin® ge Toronto, or Humalog® insulin, you must wait at least two days before making any new adjustment. On the other hand, if the adjustment involves long-acting insulin (Humulin® U, Novolin® ge Ultralente), you must wait at least three days before making any new change of any insulin dose (whether long-acting, short-acting or rapid-acting). **The only one exception to this rule is if you have two consecutive hypoglycemic readings in the same period of the day. In such a case, ignore this rule and reduce the insulin dose.** In case of hypoglycemia or hyperglycemia, do not wait more than one week to adjust the appropriate insulin dose.

10. In the "premixed" insulin regimens, which blood glucose level is affected by each insulin mixture injected?

Which insulin:	will affect the blood glucose level:
The rapid-acting[a] or short-acting[b] and intermediate-acting insulin before breakfast ➡	lunch and dinner
The rapid-acting[a] or short-acting[b] and intermediate-acting insulin before dinner ➡	bedtime and breakfast

[a] *Humalog® Mix 25*
[b] *For example, Humulin® 30/70, Novolin® ge 30/70*

The blood glucose level at any given time always reflects the effect of the **preceding** insulin dose injected.

11. How should insulin doses be adjusted in "premixed" regimens?

In general, in case of **hypoglycemia (blood glucose level below 4 mmol/L)**, as defined in the golden rules, at bedtime and in the morning, or before lunch and dinner, the dose of the appropriate premixed insulin should be reduced by two units at a time. However, if the total daily dose of insulin is less than or equal to 20 units, reduce the dose by only one unit at a time.

In general, in case of **hyperglycemia (blood glucose level above 7 mmol/L)**, as defined in the golden rules, at bedtime and in the morning, or before lunch and dinner, the dose of appropriate premixed insulin should be increased by two units at a time. However, if the total daily dose of insulin is less than or equal to 20 units, increase the dose by only one unit at a time.

Remember that premixed insulin affects glucose levels **at two periods of the day**. Therefore, if there is a discrepancy between the blood glucose levels at bedtime and in the morning (e.i. high at bedtime and low in the morning) or between the levels before lunch and dinner, **you must consult your doctor as this may indicate that the mixture needs to be changed**.

After any change of an insulin dose, you must wait at least two days before making another adjustment. In case of hypoglycemia or hyperglycemia do not wait more than one week to adjust the appropriate insulin dose.

12. In the "combined" regimen, which blood glucose level is affected by insulin injected at bedtime?

In the "combined" regimen, it is the **morning blood glucose level** that is affected by intermediate-acting or long-acting insulin injected at bedtime.

13. How should insulin doses be adjusted in the "combined" regimen?

In general, in case of **morning hypoglycemia (blood glucose level below 4 mmol/L)**, as defined in the golden rules, the insulin dose at bedtime should be reduced by two units at a time. However, if the dose is less than or equal to 10 units, reduce the dose by only one unit.

In general, in case of **morning hyperglycemia (blood glucose level above 7 mmol/L)**, as defined in the golden rules, the insulin dose at bedtime should be increased by two units at a time. However, if the dose is less than or equal to 10 units, increase the dose by only one unit.

After any change of an insulin dose, you must wait at least two days before making any new adjustment. In case of hypoglycemia or hyperglycemia, do not wait more than one week to adjust the appropriate insulin dose.

Notes

Notes

Chapter 20
Physical activities

1. Why is regular physical activity important?

When practised on a regular basis, physical activity provides the following benefits:

1) **improves physical fitness**;

2) **improves psychological well-being**;

3) **reduces the risk of heart and circulatory diseases**;

4) **improves blood pressure**;

5) **reduces the risk of osteoporosis and arthritis**;

6) **helps to control body weight**.

2. What are the benefits of a regular exercise program to someone with diabetes?

In addition to the benefits mentioned above, a program of regular physical activities helps people with diabetes to **improve the control of their blood glucose** by increasing the sensitivity of the body to insulin.

3. What are the criteria of a good physical fitness program to help control diabetes?

A good fitness program should meet the following three criteria:

1) the exercises should be **moderate** (e.g. walking, bicycling);

2) the exercises should be done **most days of the week**;

3) you should complete a total of **30 minutes of physical activity every day**.

  ■ The physical activity can be done in small periods at a time to promote greater expenditure of energy; we benefit from physical activity if we increase energy expenditure.

4) Health Canada recommends that you combine exercises that develop endurance, muscular strength and flexibility.

Types of exercises

Endurance exercises:
Sustained activities that make your heart and lungs work.

Dancing	Walking	Skating	Cross-country skiing
Golf (without a cart)	Swimming	Snowshoeing	Bicycling

Exercises for developing muscular strength:
Activities using weights or resistance to strengthen the muscles and bones and to improve posture.

Muscle development with weights or mechanical devices	Sit-ups	Sawing/ stacking wood	Carrying shopping bags

Exercises for flexibility:
Stretching, bending and light extension to relax the muscles and stay supple.

Curling	Golf	Vacuuming	Tai Chi
Dancing	Gardening	Bowling	Yoga

For a person weighing 60 kg, moderate activity is defined as one inducing the expenditure of 4.5 calories per minute. The energy expenditure must be higher for someone heavier, and must be less for someone lighter. All physical activity programs should be started gradually.

4. How much energy is expended by different physical activities?

The energy expended by various physical activities by a person weighing 60 kg is shown below. Remember that the intensity of any physical activity depends on the individual's physical condition.

Activities	Calories expended per minute	Activities	Calories expended per minute
Normal walking	4.5	Stationary bicycle	7.5
Cleaning windows	4.6	Rowing	7.8
Ice skating	5.3	Swimming laps in a pool	8.5
Mowing the lawn	5.5	Cross-country skiing	9.0
Badminton	6.0	Stair climbing	10.0
Bicycling on a level surface	7.0	Squash/racketball	12.0

5. What exercises are rated as light, moderate and intense?

Light	Moderate	Intense
Light housework	Mowing the lawn	Shoveling
Walking	Shopping	Foot racing
Golf (with a cart)	Golf (carrying clubs)	Cross-country skiing
Slow ice-skating	Slow jogging	Soccer
Bathing	Swimming (laps in a pool)	Hockey
Bowling	Tennis	Basketball
Social dancing	Aerobic dancing	Racketball
	Bicycling	
	Downhill skiing	

Do not go swimming or take long walks when you are alone.

6. How should you evaluate your physical condition before starting a program of moderate physical activity?

Look for signs and symptoms that might be linked to problems with your heart, circulation, eyes and nerves.

In general, **walking** is the most accessible, least dangerous and least expensive exercise. Don't walk faster than you can while keeping up a conversation.

7. Which exercises are contra-indicated?

There are circumstances when certain exercises may be contra-indicated, especially those that are vigorous:

1) if your **diabetes is poorly controlled** and if your blood glucose level is elevated (above 14 mmol/L with ketone bodies

in the urine, or above 17 mmol/L with or without ketone bodies in the urine). In such situations, exercise raises the level of catecholamines (if there is a lack of insulin, these hormones raise the blood glucose level and ketone bodies);

2) if you have **heart problems**, choose a supervised exercise program;

3) in case of **eye problems** with the risk of hemorrhage, **avoid** boxing, weight lifting, exercises with rapid head movements, and exercise with jarring impact on the body (including jogging and racket sports); also, avoid playing the trumpet. **Instead, practise swimming, walking, or stationary bicycling**;

4) if you have **severe neurological problems** involving complete loss of sensation in the feet, avoid the treadmill, long walks, jogging and any exercises that involve jumping. **Instead, practise swimming, bicycling, rowing, arm exercises and exercises performed while sitting**;

Remember: **Walking** is almost always permissible, even in these special cases.

8. What are the potential dangers of exercise for people with diabetes treated with oral antidiabetic medications or insulin?

Exercising increases the body's sensitivity to insulin. People with diabetes treated with oral medications of the sulfonylurea or meglitinide type, or insulin, risk **hypoglycemia, especially if the exercise is unplanned, moderate and prolonged**.

Don't forget that moderate exercise extending over several hours (e.g. cross country skiing) **can cause delayed hypoglycemia up to 12-16 hours after the physical activity.** The same effect (late hypoglycemia) can be produced by cleaning the house or spending half a day shopping.

Insulin will be absorbed faster if the **injection site** is in a part of the body to be actively used in the exercise (e.g. the thigh before fast walking, or the arm before tennis). To avoid this problem, inject insulin into the abdomen instead.

■ Be sure to check the **condition of your feet** before and after exercise.

■ Do not consume **alcohol** before, during or after exercise.

■ Always wear a **bracelet or pendant** identifying you as a diabetic.

9. How can hypoglycemia be prevented during exercise or physical activity?

To prevent hypoglycemia from occurring when you engage in exercise or physical activity, observe the following rules:

1) **plan** the day and time of the exercise (e.g. a fast-paced walk two hours after a meal on Monday, Wednesday and Friday) and, if recommended by the care team, **reduce your insulin doses** before the exercise;

2) **always measure your capillary blood glucose level** before, during and after exercise. You should also monitor it more often in the 24 hours following prolonged exercise;

3) increase your **intake of carbohydrates if the exercise is not planned**.

People with diabetes who exercise regularly need less insulin and are therefore less susceptible to hypoglycemia during exercise, even when it is not planned. People with diabetes who rarely exercise need more insulin and are therefore more susceptible to hypoglycemia after even a small amount of unplanned exercise.

10. When does exercise call for additional food?

A person with diabetes treated only with diet generally does not need to take an additional snack. However, it is important to drink enough water to have adequate fluid intake.

A person with diabetes **treated with oral antidiabetic medications such as sulfonylureas or meglitinides, or who injects insulin, may have to take an additional snack before undertaking a physical activity**:

1) if the exercise is unplanned;

2) if the blood glucose level is **below 5.5 mmol/L**:

   ■ take enough carbohydrates during the exercise to avoid hypoglycemia;

   ■ you can determine the quantity of carbohydrates you need to consume and how often to snack according to the blood glucose results obtained during the different exercise sessions. Be careful, do not overconsume!

3) It is sometimes necessary to **add carbohydrates** to the usual evening snack to protect against the prolonged effects of exercising.

11. By how much should the pre-meal dose of short-acting or rapid-acting insulin be reduced if exercise is to start one to two hours after eating?

The reduction of short-acting or rapid-acting insulin depends on the intensity and length of the exercise you will be doing after the meal:

Intensity	Reduction* in the insulin dose for exercise lasting	
	30 minutes	60 minutes
Light exercise	25%	50%
Moderate exercise	50%	75%
Intense exercise	75%	100%

* The suggested reduction is given for guidance; it should be adjusted for each person.

Notes

Notes

Chapter 21
Diabetic acidosis and the hyperosmolar state

1. What is diabetic acidosis?

Diabetic acidosis is a condition characterized by a buildup of ketone bodies in the blood, which makes the blood acidic and causes **excessive fatigue, nausea, vomiting and sometimes abdominal pain**. It also gives the breath a fruity odor, causes intense thirst, deep and rapid breathing, and a change in mental state resulting in confusion and sometimes **coma** that can be fatal.

Diabetic acidosis occurs mostly in individuals with type 1 diabetes, but in certain stressful situations, it can affect people with type 2 diabetes.

2. What is the cause of diabetic acidosis?

Diabetic acidosis is **always** caused by a **lack of insulin** in the blood. When insulin is lacking, glucose cannot enter the body's cells and accumulates in the blood. The body is then forced to get energy from its fat reserves. The **breakdown of fat** produces acidic ketone bodies which build up in the blood and spill over into the urine.

This complication of diabetes may occur if you **forget** your insulin injections or miscalculate the dosage.

Diabetic acidosis is sometimes caused by an **increased need for insulin** (e.g. when you are sick, have an infection, are under significant stress or are taking certain medications, such as cortisone).

3. How can diabetic acidosis be detected?

Diabetic acidosis may be detected by the **presence of ketone bodies** in the urine or in the blood, along with a high capillary blood glucose level, often higher than **20 mmol/L**.

4. How can diabetic acidosis be avoided?

In general, diabetic acidosis can be avoided by taking the following precautions:

1) Regularly check your capillary blood glucose level and, if indicated, check your urine for the presence of ketone bodies. Do these **tests more often** when you are sick, under significant stress, and especially if your capillary blood glucose level is **higher than 15 mmol/L**.

2) Follow the **meal plan** recommended by your dietitian.

3) Take your prescribed **insulin** dosage.

4) Follow the **recommendations** of your doctor and dietitian concerning your **diet** (solid food and liquids) and the **insulin doses** to inject if any illness makes it difficult to eat normally.

5) **Call your doctor or go to emergency in any one of these four situations**:

   - your level of **ketone bodies is moderate (4 mmol/L) to high (16 mmol/L)**;

   - your **capillary blood glucose level is higher than 20 mmol/L**;

- **you are vomiting continuously and cannot hold down liquids**;

- the **following conditions persist** despite treatment: excessive fatigue, abdominal pain, nausea and vomiting, breath with a fruity odor, intense thirst, deep and rapid breathing.

To summarize

Appropriate action should be decided on:

1) the capillary blood glucose level

2) the presence or absence of ketone bodies in urine

3) the presence or absence of signs and symptoms

blood glucose levels (mmol/L)	Ketone bodies in urine*	Symptoms**	Suggested actions
13 – 15	- or +	+	Measure your blood glucose level every 6 hours Drink 250 mL of water every hour Adjust your insulin accordingly Contact your doctor
15 – 20	++ or +++	++ or +++	Measure your blood glucose level every 4 hours Drink 250 mL of water every hour Adjust your insulin accordingly Contact your doctor Go to the hospital if there is no improvement and/or if symptoms of diabetic acidosis appear
>20	- or +++ or ++++	++++	Go to the hospital

* + = traces = 0.5 mmol/L
++ = small = 1.5 mmol/L
+++ = moderate = 4.0 mmol/L
++++ = large = 8.0-16.0 mmol/L

** + = polyurea + polydipsia
++ = diarrhea and nausea
+++ = nausea, vomiting and diarrhea
++++ = nausea, vomiting, diarrhea, with or without ketone bodies

5. What is a hyperosmolar state?

A hyperosmolar state may occur particularly in a type 2 diabetic who develops **resistance to insulin**. Due to this resistance to insulin, glucose does not properly enter the cells of the body and accumulates in the blood.

If kidney function is slightly impaired, it is more difficult to eliminate excess blood glucose through the urine. As a result, blood glucose can reach extremely high levels (**more than 35 mmol/L**), especially if the person is not drinking enough fluids. However, the small amount of insulin in the blood is enough to prevent the breakdown of fat and, in general, there is no diabetic acidosis associated.

Thus, the blood glucose level rises and the person feels very tired, is thirsty (although some elderly people feel no thirst), urinates frequently and profusely, leading to dehydration. This may be followed by a drop in blood pressure and a change in mental state that can lead to confusion, **coma** and sometimes even death.

6. What causes the hyperosmolar state?

The hyperosmolar state is always caused by a **lack of insulin** in the blood.

This complication of diabetes may develop if you **forget** to take your antidiabetic medications.

The hyperosmolar state is sometimes caused by an **increased need for insulin** (e.g. when you are sick, have an infection, are under significant stress or are taking certain medications, such as cortisone).

Most of the time, the hyperosmolar state occurs in people **who do not feel thirst** or who cannot drink fluids by themselves, as is sometimes the case with elderly people or individuals who are unable to look after themselves.

7. How can the hyperosmolar state be detected?

The hyperosmolar state is manifested in general by **intense thirst**, and **frequent and profuse urination**. A blood glucose level above **20 mmol/L** is usual. In general, ketone bodies are absent in the urine.

8. How can the hyperosmolar state be avoided?

Generally, you can avoid the hyperosmolar state by observing the following advice:

1) **Drink enough fluids** if your blood glucose level is high or if a high blood glucose level is making you urinate more frequently and profusely.

2) **Check your blood glucose level regularly**, and even more often when you are ill or under significant stress.

3) **Follow the meal plan** recommended by your dietitian.

4) **Take the antidiabetic medications** that you have been prescribed.

5) **Follow the recommendations** of your doctor and dietitian concerning your diet (solid foods and liquids) and the **antidiabetic medications** to be taken when illness makes it impossible to eat normally.

Notes

Notes

Chapter 22
Chronic complications

1. What are the long-term complications associated with diabetes?

After several years, if the blood glucose level is high most of the time, complications can develop affecting:

> 1) the **eyes**;
>
> 2) the **kidneys**;
>
> 3) the **nervous system**;
>
> 4) the **heart** and **blood vessels**.

2. How can diabetes affect the eyes?

Over time, hyperglycemia can result in **changes in the small blood vessels in the eyes**, which may interfere with blood circulation and cause hemorrhaging. This condition is called **retinopathy**. If diabetes and retinopathy are not treated adequately, they can lead to loss of eyesight.

3. How can you know if your eyes have been affected by diabetes?

If the eyes are affected, you may see **spider webs** or spots in your field of vision. Consult an **ophthalmologist**, a doctor who specializes in eye diseases.

However, changes in your eyes may appear without causing impaired vision. This is why **it is important to consult an ophthalmologist regularly**.

If you have type 1 diabetes, you should consult an ophthalmologist five years after the initial diagnosis, and every two years after that. If you have type 2 diabetes, consult an ophthalmologist as soon as you are diagnosed, and every two years after that. However, with either type 1 or type 2 diabetes, if your eyes show signs of being affected by diabetes, consult an ophthalmologist every year – or more often, if necessary.

Your eyesight may undergo temporary changes (blurred vision) due to changing blood glucose levels. **Both hyperglycemia and hypoglycemia can cause blurred vision.** This problem is corrected by normalizing the blood glucose level.

4. How can you protect your eyes?

To protect your eyes:

1) **keep your blood glucose level as close to normal as possible**;

2) **consult an ophthalmologist regularly**.

5. What long-term effect can diabetes have on the kidneys?

Over the long term, hyperglycemia can cause **changes in the small blood vessels of the kidney**, interfering with their filtering and purifying functions. This condition is called **nephropathy**. If your diabetes is not well-controlled, it may lead to a complete loss of kidney function. The patient must then be treated by dialysis (artificial kidney) or undergo a kidney transplant.

6. How can you know if your kidneys have been affected by diabetes?

The effect of diabetes on the kidneys is detected by laboratory tests, the earliest sign being the presence of **microalbuminuria** (small amounts of albumin) in the urine. A rise in blood pressure can also signal the onset of damage to the kidneys.

7. How can you protect your kidneys?

To protect your kidneys:

1) **keep your blood glucose level as close to normal as possible**;

2) **have your blood pressure checked regularly**;

3) **have lab tests done once a year to check for albumin in your urine**.

8. What long-term effect can diabetes have on your nerves?

Over time, hyperglycemia can cause **damage to the nerves**, especially in the extremities (feet and toes), but also in the genitals, stomach and intestines. This condition is called **neuropathy**.

9. How can you know if your nerves have been affected by diabetes?

In most cases, you can tell when **your extremities become less sensitive to pain, heat and cold**. Another sign is a tingling or burning sensation. The diagnosis will be confirmed by your doctor or by a special test called "electromyography" (EMG).

In men, **sexual function can also be affected**. This is called **erectile dysfunction**.

When the nerves of the stomach are affected, emptying of the stomach slows down. This condition is called **gastroparesis**. Its usual signs are a bloated feeling and/or regurgitation after meals. This irregular absorption of food can be responsible for poor control of the blood glucose level (hyperglycemia and hypoglycemia.) The diagnosis is confirmed by a gastric emptying test.

When diabetes affects the intestinal nerves, there may be constipation, sometimes alternating with diarrhea.

10. What is the biggest danger when nerves in the extremities are affected?

The major danger from losing sensitivity, especially in the feet, is **injuring yourself** (through poorly-fitting shoes, hot water, a needle, etc.) **without realizing it**. Such an injury can become infected and, if your blood circulation is impaired, it can lead to **gangrene** and **amputation**.

11. How can you prevent nerve problems and their complications?

To prevent nerve problems and their complications:

1) **keep your blood glucose level as close to normal as possible**;

2) take measures to **avoid traumatizing or burning your feet**;

3) **inspect your feet daily**;

4) **consult a doctor if you have even the slightest lesion**;

5) **report any problem with your digestion**;

6) **tell your doctor about any erectile dysfunction**.

12. How can diabetes affect the heart and blood vessels?

Diabetes can affect the heart and blood vessels by accelerating the process of **arteriosclerosis**, that is, the thickening and hardening of the arteries. This can result in blockage of the circulation in certain parts of the body, such as the heart, lower limbs, and even the brain.

13. What are the possible dangers of arteriosclerosis on the heart and blood vessels?

The dangers of arteriosclerosis depend on which part of the body is affected:

1) heart ➡ **myocardial infarction** (heart attack);

2) brain ➡ **paralysis**;

3) lower limbs ➡ **limping**.

14. How can you tell if your heart and blood vessels have been affected by diabetes?

Certain signs may reveal the presence of arteriosclerosis:

1) **slow healing**;

2) **chest pain during exertion**;

3) **pain in the calves while walking** (limping).

However, arteriosclerosis may present no symptoms, especially in its early stages. It can be diagnosed only through a medical examination or special tests such as electrocardiograms (at rest and during exercise), abdominal X-ray (to look for vessel calcification), Doppler test, etc.

15. How can you prevent your heart and blood vessels from being affected by diabetes?

To reduce the risk of problems with your heart and blood vessels:

1) **keep your blood glucose as close to normal as possible**;

2) **have your blood pressure checked regularly**;

3) **as much as possible avoid eating saturated fats**, especially of animal origin;

4) have your lipid levels checked regularly;

5) **stop smoking (if applicable)**.

Notes

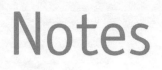

Notes

Chapter 23

Foot care

1. Why should people with diabetes take special care of their feet?

The feet of people with diabetes require special care since they are more fragile than the feet of non-diabetic people. Indeed, over the long-term, hyperglycemia can result in the following problems affecting the feet:

1) damaged **nerves** with loss of sensitivity to pain, heat and cold;

2) a **tendency for the skin to be thinner and dryer**, to become irritated more easily, and to form corns at pressure points on the feet;

3) a **tendency for the arteries to thicken and harden**, thereby compromising circulation in the feet;

4) weakened defense against germs in case of **microbial infection**.

2. How can you reduce the risks of problems to your feet?

To limit the risks of foot problems:

1) control your blood glucose level properly;

2) stop smoking (if applicable);

3) lose weight, if necessary;

4)   reduce your consumption of alcohol (if applicable);

5)   exercise regularly;

6)   see a podiatrist or a nurse experienced in foot care, if necessary.

3. What are the ten commandments of foot care for people with diabetes?

The ten commandments of foot care for people with diabetes are:

1)   **Inspect** your feet every day. If need be, ask for help from someone close to you.

2)   **Never walk barefoot** – not even in the house, and especially not on the beach.

3)   **Wash your feet every day with soap and lukewarm water.** With a thermometer, check that the water temperature is less than 35°C. Avoid prolonged foot baths. Dry your feet carefully, especially between the toes (a hair dryer can be useful).

4)   **If your skin is very dry**, apply a neutral moisturizing cream. Use a pumice stone to rub zones of hyperkeratosis, that is where the skin is thickened.

5)   **Keep your nails sufficiently long**, and file them instead of cutting them -- this is important to prevent them from penetrating the skin (ingrown toenails).

6)   **Never treat calluses, corns or blisters yourself**. Do not practise "bathroom surgery" (e.g. by removing a corn with a razor blade)! Inform your podiatrist or foot care nurse that you are diabetic. Do not use corn removers or other strong products (e.g. Parisienne® or other bleaches).

7) **Change your socks every day.**

8) **Choose proper shoes:** Your shoes should be soft and big enough. Make sure there are no foreign objects in your shoes before putting them on. Avoid very high heels. Break in new shoes gradually (wear them only a half hour per day in the beginning, for example).

9) **Be careful not to get burnt** (by hot water bottles, scalding water, sunstroke) or frostbitten.

10) **Immediately inform your doctor** about any lesion or suspicious coloration.

4. What moisturizing creams can people with diabetes use for foot care?

There are a number of moisturizing creams available for foot care, at various prices. For everyday care, a cream with a water base is recommended (e.g. Nivea®, Vaseline Intensive Care®).

5. What antiseptic products can people with diabetes use to treat a foot injury?

When a diabetic person suffers a foot injury, the cut must first be washed with soap and water, then rinsed well and dried. The cut can then be disinfected with:

1) a 70% alcohol swab;

2) a proviodine pad;

3) Hibidil® (chlorhexidine gluconate 0.05%).

If your doctor prescribes foot baths, one of the following can be added to a liter of lukewarm, boiled water:

1) 15 mL (1 tablespoon) of proviodine;

2) 15 mL (1 tablespoon) of Hibitane® 4% (chlorhexidine gluconate 4%);

3) 30 mL (2 tablespoons) of Hibitane® 2% (chlorhexidine gluconate 2%).

Rewash the foot in running water and dry well, especially between the toes. If the cut does not heal, consult your doctor.

Notes

Notes

Chapter 24
Living with diabetes

1. Why is there a psychologist on the Diabetes Day Care Unit team?

The presence of a psychologist reflects the fact that stress plays a major role in regulating your blood glucose level. As a specialist in human behavior, a psychologist can help you pinpoint sources of stress and your reactions to them, helping you work on developing attitudes and behaviors that deal with stress effectively. A comprehensive approach to the disease best helps people with diabetes to take charge of their disease.

By significantly reducing complications involving the eyes, nerves and kidneys, intensive treatment greatly improves the quality of life as well as the lifespan of people with diabetes. Remember that such treatment can bring reductions of:

- 27% to 76% of diabetic retinopathy

- 34% to 57% of nephropathy

- 60% of neuropathy

2. Why should you be concerned about stress?

Because stress triggers physiological reactions. It promotes the secretion of certain hormones that allow reserves of glucose stored in the liver to enter the bloodstream. In addition, stress reduces the effect of insulin by increasing the resistance of cells to insulin. As a result, stress can interfere with the control of blood glucose and make glucose levels increase.

3. Does stress cause diabetes?

Many patients believe that their diabetes was caused by stress. They see a connection between an unhappy experience in their life and the onset of the disease. There can be no doubt of the link between stress provoked by psychological tension and high blood glucose. However, **there is no proof that stress causes diabetes**. If the disease is latent in someone who has never shown any symptom, that person may become symptomatic after a major stressful event.

4. What are the causes of stress that are specific to diabetes?

Some forms of stress specifically linked to diabetes relate to being **in a state of denial of the disease** and the limitations it imposes on a person's **lifestyle**. Other tensions are due to fear of the long-term and short-term **complications of the disease**. These stresses create disturbances which may affect physical, psychological and social functioning.

5. How can a diabetic manage stress effectively?

Upon first hearing the diagnosis of the disease, or learning about a serious complication from it, the diabetic enters a **grieving period** over the loss of a generally good state of health. The diabetic person must begin moving towards acceptance of the disease and must learn to live with it and its unpredictability. The first thing to do is to **be aware of stress** to better manage it.

6. What is a grieving period?

Grieving refers to any situation in which you **experience a loss**. In this case, the bereavement involves your health. Grieving is essential in every painful experience of life.

You must realize that **grieving is a process that is spread over time**. Emotions provoked come and go in a disorderly manner. You may think the grieving has been resolved, when suddenly it starts all over again! Emotions surge forward once again, leading towards a higher level of acceptance.

7. How can you accept your illness?

First, by recognizing the **value of change from the negative feelings you are going through**. These feelings are there, they exist freely; in fact, they are freer than you. So you are tempted to say: "I cannot stop them!" However, you are not responsible for those feelings. Forget the philosophy of "positive thinking" which means nothing. **Negative feelings are not bad.** They are just unpleasant.

It's normal to react negatively. You need to give yourself time to become aware of these feelings. Then, you can start working on changing harmful attitudes and behaviors.

By **becoming aware** of your feelings and your reactions to them, you will be able to overcome and influence the grieving process.

You do not have control over the time you'll need to accept this.

However, you have the responsibility to become informed and to observe yourself. Unfortunately, there are no indicators for these feelings as there are for your blood glucose level.

Your **self-observation** and the confidence that you have in close friends and relatives will help you to master your feelings, attitudes and behaviors.

8. How can you identify the emotions associated with the process of grieving?

Begin by wanting to learn about the process and how to name these emotions. Then, by trying to recognize yourself in these emotions, **learn to know yourself**.

The grieving process is an **unconscious defense mechanism** aimed at adapting to reality. You do not need to think about it. It operates on its own.

9. What are the emotions involved in grieving?

There are five emotions. They exist in all of us, but not necessarily in the order presented here. They come and go in a disorderly manner:

1) **The state of negation or denial.** In this phase, you are aware of the reality of the situation but deny certain aspects that are unbearable, such as the severity of the disease or its complications. This defense mechanism helps you to avoid being overwhelmed by anxiety. Although denial may not seem very logical, it enables the psyche to eventually assimilate the full reality.

2) **The state of anger or revolt.** In this phase, you continue to deny reality, but your more or less aggressive irritation actually helps you during the process of growing more aware. Aggressiveness helps you cope with the psychological pain you feel.

3) **The state of bargaining or dealing.** In this phase, you begin to accept your situation, but your acceptance is conditional to preserve or revive your self-esteem, seriously damaged by what you perceive to be a loss of integrity.

4) **The state of depression.** In this phase, you realize that denial is useless and you feel, more dramatically, the limitations imposed by the disease. This feeds a sense of being powerless which may lead to emotional withdrawal and dependency.

5) **The state of acceptance.** In this phase, you come to a realistic, active acceptance of your illness. Taking the situation in hand helps strengthen your self-esteem and compensates for the loss of integrity.

10. Are some emotional problems more widespread among people with diabetes?

Yes. We know that depression and anxiety affect many people in the general population. However, research indicates that depression and anxiety disorders are more frequent among people with a physical illness such as diabetes.

It is estimated that depression affects people with diabetes up to three times more than the general public (20% vs. 5-10%). Similarly, anxiety disorders are up to six times more frequent (30% vs. 5%).

It is therefore important to diagnose these psychological problems since they both have a strong influence on the control of blood glucose. The more depressed or anxious you feel, the harder it is to control your diabetes.

11. What are the signs of depression?

You must first distinguish between the state of depression, which is a normal emotion associated with the process of grieving, and clinical depression, which is a disease. A depressed mood does not automatically imply a diagnosis of depression.

Depression becomes a disease when the following symptoms **have already lasted several weeks** and begin **to affect a person's work and social life**:

1) depressed, sad, hopelessness, discouraged, "at the end of my rope" feelings for most of the day, almost every day;

2) no interest in – or pleasure from – practically any activity;

3) unexplained loss of appetite or weight, or unexplained increase in appetite or weight;

4) insomnia, or the need to sleep more than usual;

5) agitation (e.g. difficulty keeping still) or slowing down of psychomotor functions (e.g. slower speech, monotone voice, long delay before answering a question, slower bodily movements, etc.);

6) lack of energy, tired feeling;

7) feelings of lost dignity, self-blame, and excessive or inappropriate guilt;

8) difficulties concentrating, thinking or making a decision;

9) recurrent thoughts of death, suicidal impulses or actual suicide attempts.

12. What should you do if you think you are suffering from depression?

If you've experienced some or many of these symptoms for two weeks or more, be sure to inform your doctor. To get appropriate help, it is important to determine if the symptoms (e.g. loss of weight, fatigue, impaired concentration) are due to your diabetes or depression.

Although the state of depression may be a normal part of the grieving process after the diagnosis of diabetes, you should consult a doctor if this condition becomes more intense and continues for several weeks.

Depression is one of the easiest mental health problems to treat, especially if it is diagnosed promptly. Most people suffering from depression can be helped by anti-depressant medication and/or psychotherapy. A combination of these two therapeutic approaches is recognized as the most effective form of treatment. Equally important is support by family, friends and support groups.

13. How can you recognize anxiety disorders?

There are mental health problems in which the major disturbance is anxiety. Phobias (e.g. phobia of needles, of low blood glucose) and generalized anxiety are the problems most frequently encountered by people with diabetes.

A diagnosis of generalized anxiety disorder may be made if these three symptoms are present at the same time:

1) anxiety and excessive worry concerning various events or activities most of the time for at least six months;

2) difficulty controlling this preoccupation;

3) intense distress.

Furthermore, at least three other symptoms among the following must also be present:

1) restlessness, feeling keyed up or on edge;

2) easily fatigued;

3) difficulty concentrating or mind going blank;

4) irritability;

5) muscular tension;

6) disturbed sleep.

14. What should you do if you think you are suffering from anxiety disorder?

If you show signs of generalized anxiety or phobia, speak to your doctor who can evaluate the situation and recommend an appropriate treatment or refer you to a mental health professional.

Anxiety disorders can be treated by medication and/or by psycho-therapy. Relaxation techniques are often employed for these conditions.

15. Where can you find help for problems of depression or anxiety disorder?

Speak to your doctor who may, in certain cases and if indicated, begin treatment with medication, and refer you to a mental health specialist, such as a psychiatrist or psychologist. These professional services are available through the public health system. You can find them in the departments of psychiatry or psychological services of hospitals or among mental health services offered by some local clinics.

You may also directly consult psychiatrists and psychologists in private practice. Obtain references by contacting appropriate professional associations.

Remember

Your personality shapes your reaction to diabetes.

While you cannot control what emotions you feel, you can control your behavior.

You cannot control how long the grieving process will take, but you have the responsibility to inform yourself and observe yourself.

You are not responsible for your illness, but you are responsible for how you manage it.

Notes

Notes

Chapter 25
Managing daily stress

1. What is stress?

Stress is defined as the **nonspecific response of the body to all demands made upon it**. Quite simply, stress is a part of life. If we didn't have stress, we'd be dead!

Indeed, we react to everything that happens to us, not only on the physical but also on the psychological, social and spiritual levels.

2. What are the causes of stress?

Stress is caused by an event that you perceive to be threatening to your well-being and beyond your capacity to deal with it. This underlies at least two conditions:

1) the importance you give to the event;

2) an imbalance between your individual capacities and the demands made by external or internal situations.

Stress can thus be provoked by external demands (surrounding pressures of your physical or social environment) or by internal demands (e.g. psychological conflict, personal crisis, attitudes).

3. What are the sources of stress?

The sources of stress are extremely varied and the stress felt depends on each individual: what may provoke stress in one person will not necessarily do so in someone else. There are three general categories of stressors.

1) **physical stressors:**

- sickness and its consequences;

- fatigue;

- pain, etc.

2) **psychological stressors:**

- emotions;

- attitudes;

- behaviors, etc.

3) **social stressors:**

- interpersonal and professional relationships;

- death of someone close;

- lifestyle changes (e.g. marriage, moving, retirement, etc.).

It should be pointed out that stress can be triggered by happy events (e.g. marriage, birth of a child, job promotion), not just unpleasant events.

4. What influences your response to stress?

Various factors influence your response to stress, including:

1) **personal factors:** personality, past experiences, attitudes, etc.

2) **emotions when facing illness:** stages of the grieving process.

3) **personal resources:** adaptation mechanisms, support, information, etc.

5. How can you recognize the symptoms of stress?

There are many indicators of stress:

1) **physical symptoms:**

- more rapid heartbeat;

- rise in blood pressure;

- increased muscular tension;

- faster breathing;

- chronic fatigue;

- headache and backache;

- tightness in the chest;

- digestive problems;

- twitching, etc.

2) **psychological symptoms:**

- aggressiveness;

- depression;

- unprovoked crying or inability to cry;

- feelings of emptiness or dissatisfaction;

- ambivalence;

- decrease in concentration, attention;

- lower motivation;

- lower self-esteem;

- nightmares, etc.

3) **behavioral symptoms:**

- irritability;

- angry outbursts;

- very critical attitude;

- forgetfulness, indecisiveness;

- lower productivity;

- increased consumption (e.g. tobacco, alcohol, food, medications) or loss of appetite;

- sexual problems, etc.

Although we are capable of dealing adequately with occasional stress, persistent, intense and frequent stress can overtax our body and produce undesirable psychological states. Since stress is an intricate part of human life, we cannot eliminate it. However, we can learn how to control it and minimize its effects.

6. How can you improve your response to stress?

First, you must recognize the symptoms of stress, then become aware that your state of stress represents a starting point. After that, you can evaluate the situation and decide on the means of action. Set simple and realistic objectives to help you realize your goal. You can gradually become aware of the full range of emotions in play and work on your personal attitudes. It is a long-term effort for personal growth.

7. What attitudes and behaviors will help a person adapt to diabetes?

1) **Manage the disease effectively:**

   ■ check your blood glucose regularly;

   ■ eat wisely and well;

   ■ engage in physical exercise;

   ■ become informed about the disease;

   ■ take good care of yourself, including relaxation.

2) **Deal with external stressors:**

   ■ manage your time well (e.g. plan, set priorities, etc.);

   ■ make changes gradually;

   ■ change your environment, if necessary;

   ■ engage in activities that bring you satisfaction;

   ■ equip yourself to handle stress (e.g. relaxation);

   ■ act as soon as possible, but in a gradual manner (not everything at once).

3) **Deal with psychological stressors:**

- control your irrational ideas or beliefs;

- keep an open mind about opinions different from your own;

- think in terms of the problem to be resolved;

- draw on social support (e.g. family, friends, support groups);

- speak to and confide in someone you trust: confiding helps you feel better;

- consult a specialist if your resources seem inadequate.

8. Should you talk about this with your close friends and relatives?

You need to realize that, like you, your family and close friends are in a state of shock, especially right after the diagnosis is made. It is very important that you talk with them openly. They are worried about you and need information to help you properly. Communication is always a winning formula. In this situation, you have a training role to play by providing those around you with general information about diabetes, how it is going to affect your lifestyle and the complications that may arise. Then, express your own needs and expectations. This is the first step towards clear mutual understanding and a measure of safety.

9. What reactions should you expect from them?

People who are closest to you usually want to help, but they don't always do it the right way. Sometimes, you may get the impression that they want to control everything and tell you what you should and shouldn't do. Or they may try to minimize the seriousness of the disease and to coax you away from strict adherence to your required regimen. The problem is often due to lack of information. So keep people informed and aware of your needs and expectations. You are in charge of your life.

10. Should you talk about it at work?

It is important to find allies. In case of emergency, these people can help you. It is your responsibility to create "a climate of safety" around you. Your success or failure in doing this will lower or increase your level of stress.

11. How can you keep up your motivation?

Motivation is an ingredient that is essential in successfully controlling your diabetes. While it is not always easy to follow these recommendations day after day, here are some ways you can help yourself:

1) adopt realistic attitudes and strive for acceptance of the disease;

2) get to know the disease well: inform yourself so that you can make clear choices;

3) demonstrate active concern: remember your health is at stake;

4) maintain a good relationship with your doctor: the two of you should work as a team;

5) set realistic goals and know how to recognize even small signs of progress;

6) experiment gradually: changing your behavior takes time;

7) accept support from other people: talking, confiding and sharing help a lot;

8) make the people around you aware of your needs: for your part, show flexibility.

9) avoid an "all-or-nothing" approach: slip-ups can occur; we're only human.

12. What does relaxation involve?

Relaxation is an important tool for controlling stress. While stress produces a number of reactions, such as stimulating many physiological functions (e.g. cardiovascular, respiratory, muscular, etc.), relaxation produces the opposite effect, thereby re-establishing physical and psychological equilibrium. Relaxation has a much deeper effect than simply "resting".

13. What relaxation exercises are easy to do?

Several techniques can be used, but two of the best-known are:

1) active relaxation, which consists of alternating tension and release;

2) passive relaxation, which consists of gradually relaxing all parts of your body in succession, while naming them mentally.

Stop your regular activity and cut yourself off from outside stimulation (e.g. noise, light, activity). Sit down, close your eyes, and breathe deeply at your own pace. After a few minutes, you will notice that your breathing has slowed down. Starting from your feet and moving upwards to your head, mentally go through each part of your body and relax it. You will soon be feeling sensations of warmth, heaviness and calm. With practice, you will be able to achieve this state of relaxation within five minutes in any location – even in public places. It's just a matter of training, and it is easy, accessible and, best of all, very effective.

14. Are there tools for promoting relaxation?

You have an interesting choice of **tape cassettes**. Experiment and discover what you prefer.

Some suggestions for beginners:

- *Progressive Relaxation and Breathing. 1987. Oakland, CA: New Harbinger Publications Inc.*

  - Jacobson's complete deep muscle technique, shorthand relaxation of muscle groups, deep breathing, etc.

- *Applied Relaxation Training. 1991. Oakland, CA: New Harbinger Publication Inc.*

  - How to relax all your muscles except those you actually need for a given activity, so that you can reduce your stress while driving, doing deskwork or walking.

You can find a variety of books on relaxation:

- You will surely find books that interest you in the library. It's up to you to choose. We particularly recommend *The Relaxation and Stress Reduction Workbook, 4th Edition*, by Martha Davis et al., published by New Harbinger Publications Inc.

Notes

Chapter 26
Sex and family planning

1. Can diabetes affect a person's sex life?

Diabetes can cause problems affecting sexuality in both men and women. The problems are less obvious in women and do not prevent them from having sexual intercourse. Women's problems in this regard have not been researched as fully as men's and less is known about them. In men, however, continually high levels of blood glucose may result in **sexual impotence**, preventing them from obtaining full satisfaction in sexual relations.

2. Do all diabetic men develop sexual impotence?

No. Men who have diabetes will not necessarily be affected by sexual impotence.

3. How can diabetes cause sexual impotence in men?

Over the long-term, hyperglycemia can cause two problems in the penis:

1) damage to nerves;

2) thickening and hardening of arteries, compromising the blood circulation.

By themselves or in combination, these two problems can result in a man being partially or completely unable to have an erection (sexual impotence).

Sexual impotence may also be due to the overall general state of health affected by poorly-controlled diabetes. In this case, proper regulation of the blood glucose level generally allows a return to normal sexual functioning.

4. Is sexual impotence in diabetic men always due to diabetes?

No. Sexual impotence in diabetic men is often related to causes that have nothing to do with diabetes itself. These causes include:

1) medications;

2) hormonal problems;

3) psychological problems.

5. How can sexual impotence be prevented in people with diabetes?

Three steps can be taken to reduce the risks of sexual impotence:

1) better control of blood glucose;

2) following your meal plan with respect to fat;

3) no smoking (if applicable).

6. How is sexual impotence assessed in men?

The following tests are performed to evaluate sexual impotence in men:

1) Doppler test of blood flow in the penis;

2) electromyography (EMG) of the penis, measuring neurological conductivity;

3) measurement of certain hormones;

4) assessment of nocturnal erection;

5) psychological evaluation, if the preceding tests are negative.

7. Can sexual impotence in diabetic men be treated?

Yes. The key is to identify the problem accurately so that appropriate treatment may be provided:

1) some cases are improved by better control of blood glucose;

2) any hormonal problem must eventually be corrected;

3) eliminate, if possible, any medication that disturbs sexual functioning;

4) for some men, taking certain medications before sexual relations induces an erection, allowing complete sexual intercourse to take place:

   - injection of prostaglandin at the base of the penis;

   - insertion of prostaglandin suppositories (Muse®) into the urethra;

   - certain medications taken orally, such as Viagra®;

   - a number of other medications are still in the development stage and should be on the market in the near future;

5) in the case of severe organic erectile dysfunction, a penile prosthetic device may be used;

6) finally, sexual therapy directed by a qualified professional often proves helpful, either by helping the diabetic person adapt to these sexual difficulties or by resolving psycho-logical conflicts causing the sexual problems.

8. Are there risks associated with pregnancy in diabetic women?

Yes. Pregnancy can pose certain risks for women with diabetes, especially if the blood glucose level is not properly controlled. There are three types of risk:

1) **risks to the mother:**

   - aggravation of diabetic complications;

   - urinary infections;

   - acidosis if she has type 1 diabetes;

   - severe hypoglycemia.

2) **risks to the baby:**

   - spontaneous miscarriage;

   - malformations;

   - death in utero;

   - premature birth;

   - hypoglycemia at birth.

3) **risks to both mother and baby:**

   - toxemia of pregnancy characterized by high blood pressure, proteins in the urine, and edema in the lower limbs.

9. How can women with diabetes prevent pregnancy-related complications?

These complications can generally be prevented. It is **essential** that the woman consult her doctor before deciding to become pregnant. It is very important to:

1) evaluate and treat complications that might worsen during pregnancy, especially those involving the eyes;

2) control blood glucose as effectively as possible to limit the risks of malformations.

Only when these concerns have been satisfactorily addressed should a diabetic woman consider becoming pregnant.

10. Does a diabetic woman run a higher risk of complications during pregnancy?

Yes. There are certain complications linked to diabetes which put her pregnancy at greater risk for:

1) cardiac insufficiency;

2) severe arterial hypertension;

3) kidney damage with severe loss of renal functioning;

4) severe damage to the eyes.

If any of these situations develop, **therapeutic interruption of pregnancy** may have to be considered.

11. What is the risk of the baby developing diabetes if one of the parents is diabetic?

If one of the parents has **type 1 diabetes**, there is a 5% risk that the offspring will develop diabetes in the long-term.

If one of the parents has **type 2 diabetes**, there is a 25% risk that the offspring will develop diabetes in the long-term.

12. What contraceptive methods are available to women with diabetes?

There are no particular methods specifically designed for diabetic women. Certain methods carry greater risk for them than for non-diabetic women. There are two types of methods:

1) **hormonal contraception:**

- **"combined"** pills containing two hormones – estrogen and progesterone. They are effective but may carry certain risks involving the blood glucose level and blood vessels.

- **"low-dose progestin"** pills which contain a small amount of progesterone. These are effective and have little impact on the blood glucose level, but their long-term action on the blood vessels is not known.

- **"high-dose progestin"** pills which contain a high dose of progesterone. These are effective and have no influence on the blood glucose level and blood vessels.

2) **mechanical contraception**

- intra-uterine devices (IUDs) are effective and present no risks of infection provided the diabetic woman controls her blood glucose level effectively.

■ localized methods, such as condoms, diaphragms and spermicides, present no risk to the diabetic woman.

The choice of method should be guided by the woman's age, the duration and level of control of diabetes, complications, whether she smokes, the number of previous pregnancies, and especially her preferences and those of her partner.

13. What methods of sterilization are available to a diabetic woman and her partner?

Sterilization is an option that should be seriously considered in the case of a woman who has been pregnant several times before, especially if diabetes-related complications are involved. The options are:

1) tubular ligation (tying the Fallopian tubes);

2) vasectomy for the partner.

14. Can hormones be taken by a diabetic woman going through menopause?

Generally, a menopausal woman with diabetes can take estrogen and/or progestational hormonal agents.

However, taking estrogens carries certain risks for women who:

1) have a history of thrombophlebitis;

2) have a history of cerebrovascular problems and who smoke;

3) have been treated for breast cancer.

Notes

Chapter 27
Research: Future outlook

Thanks to the continuing progress made in research, we are entering the new millenium with a better understanding of the causes of diabetes and its complications.

In type 1 diabetes, it appears that a change in insulin-producing pancreatic cells by environmental factors, such as a viral infection, for example, prevents the body from recognizing its own cells so that it produces antibodies to destroy them. This ability to produce antibodies against its own cells could be transmitted genetically. These antibodies can be detected five years before the disease appears.

In type 2 diabetes, two major factors intervene in the development of the disease: resistance to insulin (so that much more insulin is needed to maintain a normal blood glucose level), and a decrease in the capacity of pancreatic cells to produce insulin. In most cases, resistance to insulin occurs many years before the development of diabetes. As long as the pancreatic cells compensate by producing more insulin, the blood glucose level remains normal.

It is only when the pancreatic cells cannot compensate and the production of insulin decreases that the blood glucose level increases. In the beginning, the blood glucose level rises, especially after meals, which is called impaired glucose tolerance – this is a prediabetic stage. If the production of insulin continues to decrease, the blood glucose level will rise even further after meals, and, finally, even before meals – this is when diabetes appears. Susceptibility to insulin resistance and the decreased capacity to produce insulin are probably transmitted genetically. In addition, excess weight and physical inactivity increase insulin resistance and, thus, in genetically-susceptible people, heighten the risk of developing diabetes.

In the last decade, two large studies have definitively confirmed that the complications of diabetes are mainly related to a high blood glucose level over several years. The first study, an American-Canadian Trial (DCCT), followed 1440 patients with type 1 diabetes and was published in 1993. The second, a British study (UKPDS), was published in 1998. It was performed on 4209 type 2 diabetes patients. Both studies concluded that the diabetic, whether type 1 or type 2, must be treated aggressively and that the target should be a blood glucose level as close to normal as possible.

It is clear that this is a great challenge. However, thanks to progress in research, we can count on new pharmacological and technological developments that will help us not only to improve control of the blood glucose level, but also perhaps cure and even prevent the disease as well as its complications.

The DCCT and UKPDS studies both showed that it is difficult to achieve a normal blood glucose level. To do so in most people with diabetes, we need new medications. Several **new antidiabetic drugs** are presently being studied. There are five major categories:

1) drugs that delay the absorption of sugar at the intestinal level – GLP-1, excendin-4 and pramlintide;

2) drugs that stimulate the secretion of insulin by the pancreas – Starlix® or nateglinide;

3) drugs that enhance the effect of insulin – GI262770XT, GI262570;

4) drugs that mimic the action of insulin, such as organic vanadium compounds and selenium;

5) insulins and insulin analogues – basal long-acting insulin (glargine insulin, detemir insulin and NN344 insulin), new rapid-acting insulin (aspart insulin), inhaled insulin (Exubera®) absorbed by the lungs, and oral insulin (Oralin®) absorbed by the oral mucous membranes.

Transplantation of the pancreas is already being done with success in many Canadian centers. The two major problems are the shortage of donors and the side effects of antirejection drugs. A group of Canadian researchers in Edmonton has recently created news by using new anti-rejection drugs and, above all, by eliminating cortisone. They have succeeded in **transplanting the islets of Langerhans**, that is to say, the pancreatic cells which produce insulin. Ambulatory transplantation is done under local anesthesia via the liver, as with liver biopsy, except that a catheter is introduced in the portal vein entering the liver and the islets are injected with a syringe. The patient can then return home. Up to now, a dozen patients have successfully received transplants and the longest follow-up is about two years with normalization of the blood glucose level without insulin injection. The problem is that over 80% of the islets are lost during isolation. Thus, two and sometimes three transplantations of the islets are required before the blood glucose level can be normalized. This makes the problem of donor shortage more acute. However, improvement of the technique of isolation of the islets should partially solve this problem.

New avenues are also being explored to find, for transplantation, cells that are capable of producing and secreting insulin. **Genetic engineering** allows us to presently take liver or gut cells, for example, and program them genetically to produce insulin. Theoretically, we can take a part of the liver, isolate the cells, program them to produce insulin and then transplant them, using the technique of the Edmonton group. In this case, we will not need antirejection drugs. However, the mechanism of insulin secretion is not the same as in pancreatic cells and regulating insulin secretion in these cells can be a problem. Therefore, much more work needs to be done so that secretion occurs on demand according to the blood glucose level. Another approach, which depends on our capacity to manipulate genes, is the humanization of the islets of Langerhans from animals, which would allow us, on the one hand, to access an inexhaustable source of islets and, on the other hand, eliminate the need for antirejection drugs. All these dreams are possible.

A major challenge for research lies in the **prevention of diabetic complications**. Thanks to our better understanding of the physio-pathological mechanisms responsible for diabetic complications, some studies are currently evaluating certain drugs that could prevent the complications of diabetes independently of the control of blood glucose. We have already emphasized the major role played by a high glucose level in the development of diabetic complications. Several studies have shown that an elevated blood glucose level is associated with the overproduction of an enzyme known as protein kinase C. Several studies have reported that this enzyme is involved in the development of complications. The pharmaceutical industry has perfected an inhibitor of protein kinase C, and it has shown that this drug can prevent complications in diabetic animals. Studies in humans are presently in progress. One such drug may eventually prevent the development of complications despite the difficulty in achieving optimal control of blood glucose.

The ultimate goal of research is the **prevention of disease**, including diabetes.

We know that in type 1 diabetes the pancreatic cells that produce insulin are destroyed by antibodies. We can measure the appearance of these antibodies about five years before the development of the disease. Some studies are investigating, in high risk groups, the possibility of preventing the disease by treatments that block the production of antibodies as soon as they appear. One study is evaluating the effect of nicotinamide on the development of type 1 diabetes. Two studies are currently looking at the effect of insulin administration either by injection or inhalation. Although preliminary results are encouraging, it is still too early to draw any conclusions.

As for type 2 diabetes, we know that the disease is preceded by a "prediabetic phase" called impaired glucose tolerance. It is possible to easily identify this prediabetic phase. A Finnish study has shown that diet and exercise reduce the occurrence of type 2 diabetes by 58% in a population presenting impaired glucose tolerance. Two other major studies are in progress. One, the "STOP-NIDDM Trial," is international, but coordinated by Canada. It is investigating the effect of acarbose. The other, "The Diabetes Prevention Program," is American. It is studying the effect of diet and exercise as well as metformin on the occurrence of diabetes in a high risk population. Another Canadian study, "the DREAM Study," on the effect of ramipril and rosiglitazone in the prevention of type 2 diabetes, began in 2001. There is much hope on the horizon.

All these research efforts at the international level, where numerous Canadian researchers are actively participating, bring much hope to people with diabetes.

Notes

Lexicon

Antidiabetic medications: Medications that lower the blood glucose level.

"Bad cholesterol": This is LDL-cholesterol or lipoproteins of low density (low-density lipoproteins). LDLs accumulate cholesterol in the walls of arteries. The saturated fatty acids and trans fatty acids in food increase the level of LDL-cholesterol.

Blood glucose: The blood sugar level.

Capillary blood glucose: The level of sugar present in a drop of blood drawn from the tip of a finger.

Carbohydrates: A general term used to designate all sugars found in foods: starch, fructose, glucose, lactose, fiber, etc.

Dietary cholesterol: A fat substance, of animal origin only, that is found in giblets, egg yolk, meat, poultry, fish, milk-based products. Excessive intake carries the risk of increasing the blood cholesterol level.

Dietary fiber: Vegetable substances not digested by the stomach or intestine.

Fatty acids: These are substances composed of fats. They may be monounsaturated, polyunsaturated, or saturated.

Glucose: Sugar.

Glucagon: A hormone that is injected, like insulin, and which raises the blood glucose level.

"Good cholesterol": This is HDL-cholesterol or lipoproteins of high density (high-density lipoproteins). HDLs transport cholesterol to the liver, where it is eliminated from the body.

Hydrogenation: A process used to harden an oil, giving it a "buttery" consistency. The procedure creates the formation of saturated fatty acids and trans fatty acids.

Hyperglycemia: Elevation of the blood glucose level above normal.

Hypoglycemia: Decrease of the blood glucose level below normal.

Kilocalories and kilojoules: These are two different units measuring the value of energy in foods: 1 kilocalorie = 4,184 kilojoules.

Monounsaturated fatty acids: Fats that are in liquid form at room temperature and found in significant amounts in olive oil, canola oil and almonds.

Polyunsaturated fatty acids: Fats that are in liquid form at room temperature and found in significant amounts in corn oil, soya oil and sunflower oil.

Proteins: Substances that contribute to the composition of body tissues (e.g. muscle, skin, hair, etc.). They are also found in different foods, such as milk products, meats and alternatives.

Saturated fatty acids: Fats that are solid at room temperature, especially those of animal origin. They are also found in certain vegetables, such as coconut oil, palm oil or in hydrogenated vegetable oils. Their presence in significant quantities in food is associated with high levels of cholesterol in blood.

Sulfonylureas: Medications that stimulate the pancreas to produce more insulin.

Trans fatty acids: Fatty acids formed during partial or total hydrogenation of oils. They seem to exert an undesirable effect on the level of cholesterol similar to the effect of saturated fatty acids.

Triglycerides: Name given to fats that we eat and to body fat. A small fraction only is found in the blood circulation. A high level of triglycerides is a risk factor for cardiovascular diseases. A diet rich in fats, carbohydrates and alcohol increases the level of triglycerides.

Type 1 diabetes: Insulin-dependent diabetes.

Type 2 diabetes: Non-insulin-dependent diabetes.

Vitamins: Elements essential for the proper functioning of the body. Among other things, they help in the use of energy, but do not provide energy.

Notes

Annexes
Golden rules for the adjustment of insulin doses

A) "Split-mixed" insulin regimen

An injection of intermediate-acting insulin (e.g. Humulin® N, Novolin® ge NPH) and rapid-acting insulin (Humalog®) or short-acting insulin (Humulin® R, Novolin® ge Toronto) before breakfast and dinner.

1. What is the desired blood glucose level?

Between 4 and 7 mmol/L before meals and at bedtime (before snack, if any).

2. Which insulin must be adjusted?

Insulin	affects	the blood glucose level before
Intermediate-acting before dinner	➡	breakfast
Rapid-acting or short-acting before breakfast	➡	lunch
Intermediate-acting before breakfast	➡	dinner
Rapid-acting or short-acting before dinner	➡	bedtime

3. Should the insulin dose be increased or decreased?

1) **Increase** the appropriate insulin dose if there is **hyperglycemia**.

2) **Decrease** the appropriate insulin dose if there is **hypoglycemia**.

4. How many units should you adjust for the dose?

1) Two units at a time if the total daily dose of insulin (intermediate-acting + rapid-acting or short-acting) is higher than 20 units.

2) One unit at a time if the total daily insulin dose (intermediate-acting + rapid-acting or short-acting) is less than or equal to 20 units.

5. What rules should be followed?

Take the time to analyze your blood glucose when calculating the average of the **last three blood glucose levels** for each period of the day (breakfast, lunch, dinner and bedtime) without going back more than seven days. Take into account only those measurements recorded since the last adjustment.

1) When calculating the average, do not use measurements less than 4 mmol/L or higher than 7 mmol/L associated with a **situation** that is **sporadic**, **exceptional** and **explainable**.

2) **Never modify** the insulin dose based on **a single blood glucose level**.

3) Always adjust **a single insulin dose at a time**, at only one period of the day.

4) Begin by correcting the **hypoglycemia** starting with the first of the day. A hypoglycemic situation is present when:

- the average is lower than 4 mmol/L for a given period of the day, or

- even if the average is higher than 4 mmol/L for a given period of the day, you find three hypoglycemias during the last seven days, or two hypoglycemias in the last two measurements.

Give a value of 2 mmol/L to all non-measured hypoglycemias.

Hypoglycemia that occurs outside the four usual blood glucose measurement periods should be entered in the next period.

5) Then, correct the **hyperglycemia** situation, which is an average higher than 7 mmol/L in a given period of the day. Begin with the first hyperglycemia of the day, then the second, etc.

6) Allow a **waiting period** of at least two days after a dose adjustment before readjusting any insulin dose.

B) "Prandial-bedtime" insulin regimen

An injection of rapid-acting insulin (Humalog®) or short-acting insulin (Humulin® R, Novolin® ge Toronto) before each meal and an injection of intermediate-acting insulin (e.g. Humulin® N, Novolin® ge NPH) at bedtime.

1. What is the desired blood glucose level?

Between 4 and 7 mmol/L before meals and at bedtime (before snack, if any).

2. Which insulin must be adjusted?

Insulin	affects	the blood glucose level before
Intermediate-acting before bedtime	➡	breakfast
Rapid-acting or short-acting before breakfast	➡	lunch
Rapid-acting or short-acting before lunch	➡	dinner
Rapid-acting or short-acting before dinner	➡	bedtime

3. Should the insulin dose be increased or decreased?

1) **Increase** the appropriate insulin dose if there is **hyperglycemia**.

2) **Decrease** the appropriate insulin dose if there is **hypoglycemia**.

4. How many units should you adjust for the dose?

1) Two units at a time if the total daily insulin dose (intermediate-acting + rapid-acting or short-acting) is higher than 20 units.

2) One unit at a time if the total daily insulin dose (intermediate-acting + rapid-acting or short-acting) is less than or equal to 20 units.

5. What rules should be followed?

Take the time to analyze your blood glucose when calculating the average of the **last three blood glucose levels** for each period of the day (morning, noon, evening and bedtime) without going back more than seven days. Only take into account the measurements obtained since the last adjustment.

1) When calculating the average, do not use measurements less than 4 mmol/L or higher than 7 mmol/L associated with a **situation** that is **sporadic**, **exceptional** and **explainable**.

2) **Never modify** the insulin dose based on a **single blood glucose level**.

3) Always adjust **a single insulin dose at a time**, at only one period of the day.

4) Begin by correcting the **hypoglycemia** starting with the first of the day. A hypoglycemic situation is present when:

   ■ the average is less than 4 mmol/L for a given period of the day, or

   ■ even if the average is higher than 4 mmol/L for a given period of the day, you find three hypoglycemias during the last seven days, or two hypoglycemias in the last two measurements.

Give a value of 2 mmol/L to all non-measured hypoglycemias.

Hypoglycemia that occurs outside the four usual blood glucose measurement periods should be entered in the next period.

5) Then, correct the **hyperglycemia** situation, which is an average higher than 7 mmol/L in a given period of the day. Begin with the first hyperglycemia of the day, then the second, etc.

6) Allow a **waiting period** of at least two days after a dose adjustment before readjusting any insulin dose.

C) "Basal-bolus" insulin regimen

An injection of long-acting insulin (Humulin® U, Novolin® ge Ultralente) at bedtime and an injection of rapid-acting insulin (Humalog®) or short-acting insulin (Humulin® R, Novolin® ge Toronto) before each meal. Premeal insulins are often given according to carbohydrate content of the meal to be ingested.

1. What is the desired blood glucose level?

Between 4 and 7 mmol/L before meals and at bedtime (before snack, if any).

2. Which insulin must be adjusted?

Insulin	affects	the blood glucose level before
Long-acting before bedtime	➡	breakfast
Rapid-acting or short-acting before breakfast	➡	lunch
Rapid-acting or short-acting before lunch	➡	dinner
Rapid-acting or short-acting before dinner	➡	bedtime

3. Should the insulin dose be increased or decreased?

1) **Increase** the appropriate insulin dose if there is **hyperglycemia**.

2) **Decrease** the appropriate insulin dose if there is **hypoglycemia**.

4. How many units should you adjust for the dose?

1) **Long-acting insulin:**

   ■ Two units at a time if the daily dose is higher than 10 units.

   ■ One unit at a time if the daily dose is less than or equal to 10 units.

2) **Rapid-acting or short-acting insulin:**

   ■ 0.2 unit/10 g of carbohydrates at a time if the dose is higher than 0.5 unit/10 g of carbohydrates.

   ■ 0.1 unit/10 g of carbohydrates at a time if the dose is less than or equal to 0.5 unit/10 g of carbohydrates.

5. What rules should be followed?

Take the time to analyze your blood glucose when calculating the average of the **last three blood glucose levels** for each period of the day (morning, noon, evening and bedtime) without going back more than seven days. Only take into account the measurements obtained since the last adjustment.

1) When calculating the average, do not use measurements less than 4 mmol/L or higher than 7 mmol/L associated with a **situation** that is **sporadic**, **exceptional** and **explainable**.

2) **Never modify** the insulin dose based on **a single blood glucose level**.

3) Always adjust **a single insulin dose at a time**, at only one period of the day.

4) Begin by correcting the **hypoglycemia** starting with the first hypoglycemia of the day. A hypoglycemic situation is present when:

   ■ the average is less than 4 mmol/L for a given period of the day, or

   ■ even if the average is higher than 4 mmol/L for a given period of the day, you find three hypoglycemias during the last seven days, or two hypoglycemias in the last two measurements.

Give a value of 2 mmol/L to all non-measured hypoglycemias.

Hypoglycemia that occurs outside the four usual blood glucose measurement periods should be entered in the next period.

5) Then, correct the **hyperglycemia** situation which is an average higher than 7 mmol/L in a given period of the day. Begin with the first hyperglycemia of the day, then the second, etc.

6) Allow a **waiting period** after adjustment before readjusting any insulin dose. Wait at least two days after changing rapid-acting or short-acting insulin. Wait at least three days after changing long-acting insulin before readjusting any insulin dose. The only exception is two consecutive hypoglycemias in the same period of the day. In such case, ignore this rule and immediately reduce the appropriate insulin.

D) "Premixed" insulin regimen

An injection of premixed insulin made from a mixture of rapid-acting or short-acting insulin and an intermediate-acting insulin (e.g. Humulin® 30/70, Novolin® ge 50/50, Humalog® Mix 25) before breakfast and dinner.

1. What is the desired blood glucose level?

Between 4 and 7 mmol/L before meals and at bedtime (before snack, if any).

2. Which insulin should be adjusted?

Premixed insulin	affects	the blood glucose level before
Rapid-acting or short-acting and intermediate-acting before breakfast	➡	lunch **and** dinner
Rapid-acting or short-acting and intermediate-acting before dinner	➡	bedtime **and** breakfast

3. Should the insulin dose be increased or decreased?

1) **Increase** the appropriate premixed insulin dose in case of **hyperglycemia**.

2) **Decrease** the appropriate premixed insulin dose in case of **hypoglycemia**.

Note: If there is a discrepancy between the blood glucose level before lunch and dinner (e.g. if it is high at lunch and low at dinner) or between the blood glucose level at bedtime or at breakfast, consult your doctor because this suggests that the mixture needs to be changed.

4. How many units should you adjust for the dose?

1) Two units at a time if the total daily premixed insulin dose is higher than 20 units.

2) One unit at a time if the total premixed insulin dose is less than or equal to 20 units.

5. What rules should be followed?

Take the time to analyze your blood glucose when calculating the average of the **last three blood glucose levels** for each period of the day (morning, noon, evening and bedtime) without going back more than seven days. Only take into account the measurements obtained since the last adjustment.

1) When calculating the average, do not use measurements less than 4 or higher than 7 mmol/L associated with a **situation** that is **sporadic**, **exceptional** and **explainable**.

2) **Never modify** the insulin dose based on a **single blood glucose level**.

3) Always adjust a **single insulin dose at a time**, at only one period of the day.

4) Begin by correcting the **hypoglycemia** starting with the first hypoglycemia of the day. A hypoglycemic situation is present when:

   ■   the average is lower than 4 mmol/L for a given period of the day, or

■ even if the average is higher than 4 mmol/L for a given period of the day, you find three hypoglycemias during the last seven days, or two hypoglycemias in the last two measurements.

Give a value of 2 mmol/L to all non-measured hypoglycemias.

Hypoglycemia that occurs outside the four usual blood glucose measurement periods must be entered in the next period.

5) Then, correct the **hyperglycemia** situations which is an average higher than 7 mmol/L in a given period of the day. Begin with the first hyperglycemia of the day, then the second, etc.

6) Allow a **waiting period** of at least two days after a dose adjustment before readjusting any insulin dose.

My personal goals

In the appropriate box, number (from 1 to 5) the goals you consider the most important to reach.

My medical follow-up	(0: Objective; N/A: Not applicable)	0	N/A
Consult my ophthalmologist regularly as recommended			
Consult my doctor at least twice a year			
Inform myself about the results of analysis and examinations performed			
Regularly check my blood pressure			
Check my microalbuminuria once a year			
Stop smoking			
Care and recommendations that I must follow			
Measure my blood glucose level, as recommended, and write the results in my personal logbook			
Measure my blood glucose level more often in case of disease			
Make sure I carry sugar with me at all times			
Wear a bracelet or pendant identifying me as a diabetic			
Check my feet every day			
Notify the **Société de l'assurance automobile du Québec (SAAQ)** about my state of diabetes (if you live in Quebec)			
My diet			
Eat the prescribed quantity of sugar with each meal			
Eat balanced meals (carbohydrates, proteins, fat)			
Choose foods rich in fiber			
Eat recommended snacks in the evening			
Eat at fixed times			
Measure my food servings at times			
Periodically update my food diary			
Choose fats that were recommended to me			
Drink alcohol only when I eat			
Perform physical exercise regularly (every day if possible)			

My medications	O	N/A
Take my medications according to my doctor's prescription		
Write in my logbook all changes in the dosage of my antidiabetic medications		
Do not change the doses of tablets, except if my doctor agrees		
Follow the "golden rules" for adjustment of my insulin doses		
Bring all my medications to each medical visit		
Ensure that non-prescription medications that I take do not affect my diabetes		
My well-being		
Identify the stress factors that particularly affect me		
Improve my reactions to stress		
Set aside at least 10 minutes a day to relax		
Speak to my family, friends and co-workers about my diabetes		
Manage my time in a way that respects my needs		

My personal goals

_____

_____

_____

_____

_____

_____

_____

_____

_____

_____

_____

_____

_____

Signature: _____ Date: _____

Targets
for optimal control

Glucose	
Glycosylated hemoglobin (HbA$_{1c}$)	< 0.070 (normal: 0.048 – 0.060)
Fasting (or before meals) blood glucose level	4 – 7 mmol/L
Blood glucose one to two hours after meals, if needed	5 – 11 mmol/L
Lipid profile	
Triglycerides	< 2 mmol/L*
LDL-cholesterol	< 2.5 mmol/L**
Total cholesterol/HDL	< 4***
Microalbuminuria	< 20 mg/min or <30 mg/24 h
Risk factors	
Blood pressure	< 130/80 mm Hg****

Height	meters:	feet:	inches:
Weight	kilos:	pounds:	
Target weight	kilos:	pounds:	
Healthy weight	< 65 years: Body mass index 20 -25	kilos:	pounds:
	> 65 years: Body mass index 25 - 27	kilos:	pounds:

Note: Treatment starts from:
*   *   *Triglycerides ≥ 2.4 mmol/L*
*   **   *LDL-cholesterol ≥ 3.0 mmol/L*
*   *** *Total cholesterol/HDL ≥ 5*
*   **** *Blood pressure ≥ 140/90 mm Hg*

My personal goals

_____

_____

_____

_____

_____

Signature: _____ Date: _____

From the same publisher

Dr. André-H. Dandavino and colleagues
The Family Guide to Health Problems (2001)

Dr. Jacques Boulay
Bilingual Guide to Medical Abbreviations, 3rd edition (1998)